Food *for* Thought

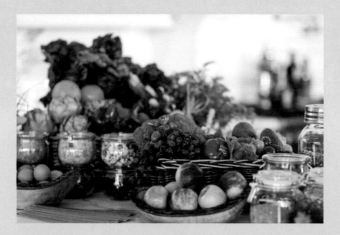

Food *for* Thought

Recipes for Ultimate Mind and Body Health

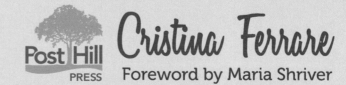

Post Hill
PRESS

Cristina Ferrare

Foreword by Maria Shriver

A POST HILL PRESS BOOK

Food for Thought:
Recipes for Ultimate Mind and Body Health
© 2018 by Cristina Ferrare
All Rights Reserved

ISBN: 978-1-64293-057-3

Cover art by Cody Corcoran

Content development, editing, interior design, and composition by
Greg Johnson/Textbook Perfect

Photography by Todd Porter and Diane Cu

Post Hill Press
New York • Nashville
posthillpress.com

Printed in China

To my friend, Maria Shriver

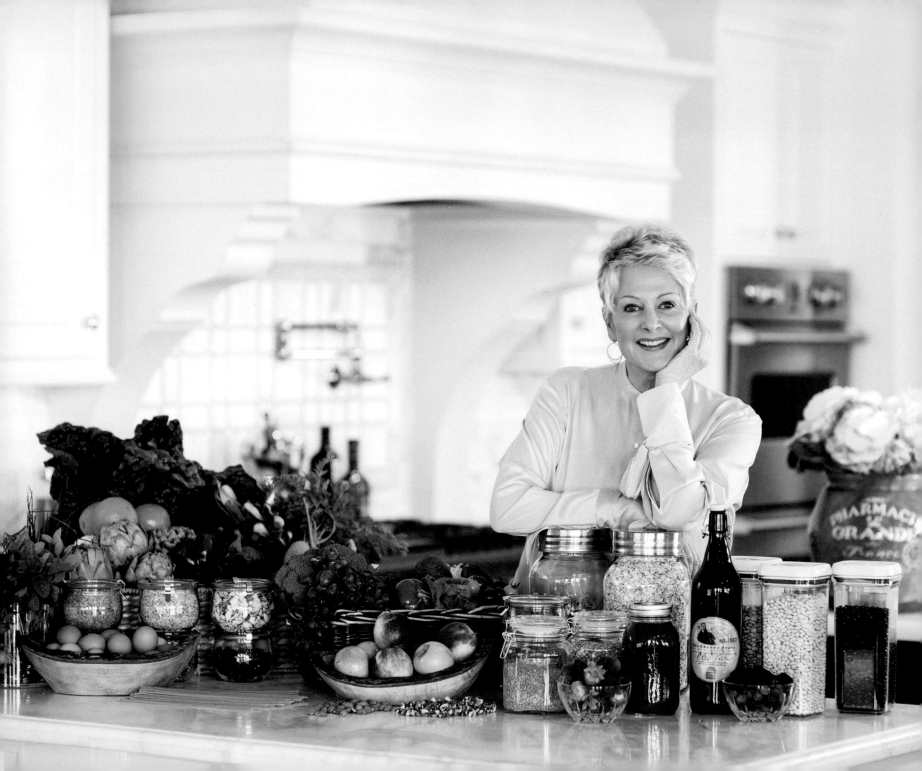

Contents

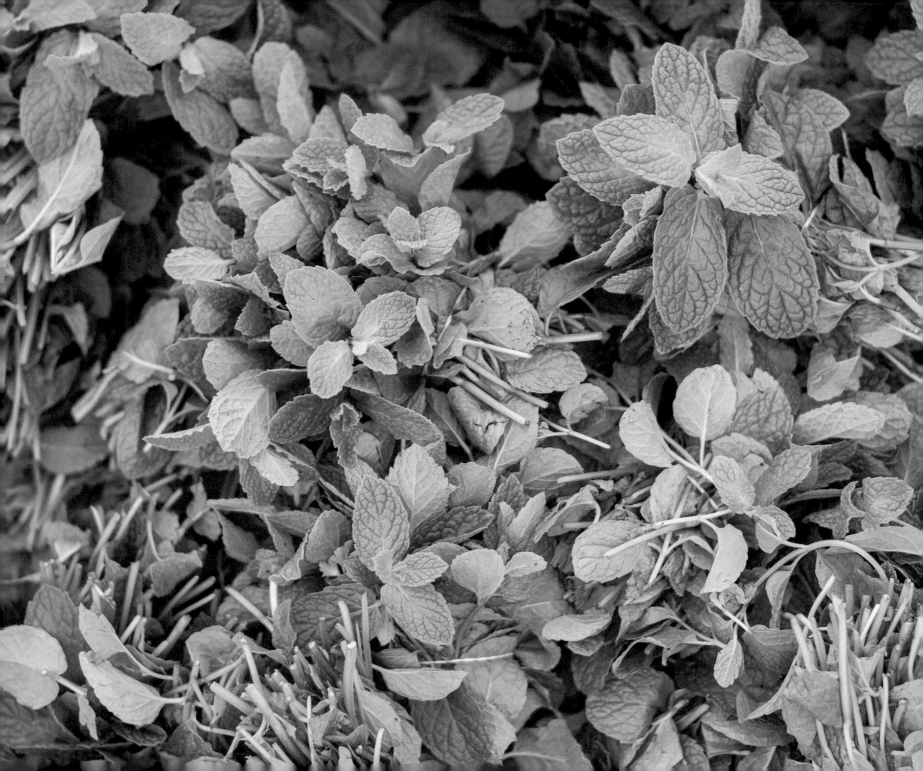

Foreword

By Maria Shriver

Wow. It's mind-blowing to me that my name is associated with a cookbook. Why? Because, as everyone close to me knows, I can't cook!

Well, it's not that I can't cook; it's just that I don't consider myself to *be* a cook. My birthday cakes are legendary, and my kids will tell you that I make a mean baked brie, but beyond that...my talents stop about there.

That said, I am a food lover. I love family dinners and just about any gathering where food brings people together. Meals have a way of nourishing more than just our bodies. They draw us closer and fill our hearts and souls.

I've always loved a good meal. I just wish that I would have known sooner how important it is to be mindful about the ingredients that go into one.

You see, I wasn't brought up understanding the impact that food has on your mind and your mood. I didn't know about the dangers of sugar. I hadn't heard about grass-fed beef or wild fish. I hadn't heard that watercress is healthier than kale. (Who knew?)

But now I do know. And now the work that I do trying to find a cure for Alzheimer's disease has led me to realize how important food is to the health of our minds. That's why I'm so thrilled to be a part of this book, which is the brainchild of my longtime friend Cristina

Ferrare. Cristina is a mind-blowing chef. Like me, she is also a child of a parent who passed from Alzheimer's. Together we are determined to do what we can to help wipe out this disease in our lifetime.

I love this cookbook because it is, in fact, food for thought. All of the recipes in here are good for you, good for your mind, and good for the world.

Why are they good for the world? Because what the world needs are healthy people with healthy minds and positive mindsets. We hope this book will inspire you to make healthier choices—ones that are good for your body and your mind.

A portion of the proceeds of this book go to The Women's Alzheimer's Movement, an organization I founded that seeks to understand why two-thirds of all the brains diagnosed with Alzheimer's in America belong to women. We're determined to answer this question, and we're also determined to educate people about the lifestyle changes they can make starting today to keep their brains working at their best.

Exercise, meditation, sleep, and cognitive training are all important to our brain health. But food is a huge component as well. Watching what you eat will not only help protect your mind in the future, but it will make you feel so much better in the here and now.

Trust me, if you follow the recipes in this book, you will feel better. You will also be doing yourself a favor by serving yourself (and the people you love) food that's healthy and good for your hearts and minds.

I hope you will join Cristina and me in our effort to inspire everyone to eat healthy, live well and protect our minds for the future. Believe me, our mind is our most precious asset. It's worth saving.

Maria

Introduction

As far back as the early 1960s the message to me was loud and clear, "You are what you eat." The brain, heart, liver, kidneys, stomach, intestines, colon, esophagus, pancreas—literally every inch of your magnificent body needs certain foods that provide nutrients to help it function, and keep your body healthy at its highest optimum.

For over forty years I have researched and written about health and the effects of food on one's health. This book is for men, women, and children!

I was given an opportunity to bring my core beliefs to the forefront through my friend Maria Shriver. Maria is a true pioneer and an outspoken advocate on issues close to her heart, to make changes that will affect people's lives and make a difference. "Moving the needle forward," as Maria likes to put it, and she is constantly doing that.

She invited me to join forces with her and her organization she founded, The Women's Alzheimer's Movement, also known as WAM. WAM raises awareness about the disproportionate effects Alzheimer's has on women, raises funds for gender-based research, educates about the connection between lifestyle and brain health, and rallies support for the 5.4 million people living with Alzheimer's and their caregivers.

Today's health statistics show among the American public both men and women, but especially women, an alarming increase in Alzheimer's disease. Every sixty-six seconds, someone will develop Alzheimer's and two-thirds of those brains belong to women—and no one knows why.

Another alarming development is the increase in heart disease, which is the #1 killer in the United States, followed by cancer (especially breast, colon, skin, and prostate cancers) and diabetes.

Both Maria and I feel passionately about research for Alzheimer's disease, finding a cure, and helping caregivers because we have had first-hand experience with this disease. Her beloved father, Sargent Shriver, and my beautiful, loving mother died of Alzheimer's.

My work with Maria gave birth to this book, *Food for Thought*. A book that is not only a cookbook but illustrates the importance of proper nutrition as a lifestyle that will enrich and, hopefully, prolong one's life while still enjoying the foods you love.

All disease begins in the gut.

—HIPPOCRATES

Starting with feeding your gut and in turn enriching your entire body, I've included recipes that are not only nutritious and delicious, but which do not deprive you of any of the foods that you enjoy.

As I did my research for this book I became acutely aware of the foods you needed to eat for gut health, along with foods you need in your diet for different parts of your body. I learned that gut health is *the* most important thing you need to fix first.

Gut health is the most important to balance because it has major effects on your brain, your moods, and your memory. The gut "talks" to your heart and brain every day and controls what goes on in your body. Some researches even refer to your gut as your "second brain."

There are so many things that can wreak havoc with our digestive systems. It is vital to your health to get things back in balance in your body to restore yourself to optimal health.

Chronic inflammation caused by foods has a serious effect on the body's inflammation responses. The biggest culprits are the processed and sugary foods and trans fats that are in a variety of snack and fried foods, sugary baked goods, and vegetable shortening. Foods that have high amounts of trans fats increase systemic inflammation.

There are numerous ways to control chronic inflammation naturally and to promote overall health, starting with your gut.

Scientists have learned how what you eat affects adult brains and the brains of children as well. It is never too early to start children on the road to body and brain health beginning with the day they are off the breast.

Omega-3 fatty acids, which you'll find in foods such as salmon, walnuts, and fruits, provide many benefits. They improve learning, aid memory, and help to fight mental disorders, such as depression, mood swings, and dementia.

Studies show that children who had increased amounts of omega-3 fatty acids perform better in school and have fewer behavioral problems.

I am convinced beyond a shadow of a doubt that what we put into our bodies directly affects our health. I use to say with gusto, *I live to eat*, but now I say, *I eat to live*. I want to participate in my life as a fully functioning human being for however long I may have. Food is now my medicine.

I've created recipes that include almost every food you can think of while eliminating white (processed) sugar, most gluten, and some dairy. However, I am realistic; even though I eat this way, most people will not give up certain things and that's okay as long as you do not make it a daily habit. You will find, however, as your body starts to feel better, your taste preference for sugary, salty, oily, and fatty foods will diminish because it won't taste good to you anymore!

I'm asking you to stop and really think from this day forward about how what you eat will affect your overall health before you put it in your mouth. You make the choice; think clearly about it so you can help your body's inflammation responses.

If you're like me, you want everybody to be happy. You want the sun to shine, people to smile, and life to be like the title of every loving, uplifting song you've ever heard. And you want everyone to be healthy.

I have come to appreciate wanting to emphasize the good things in life, even when reality sometimes crashes our dreams. So, when I was diagnosed with multiple myeloma, a cancer of the white blood cells, I vowed to fight it with a positive attitude and a heart filled with both hope and determination. I am winning that fight. I went through a stem cell replacement in 2016 and was in remission 2 months later. My doctors were amazed by how quickly I recovered! I'm convinced it is because of the choices I made in my diet, which I have been following for years, that helped me in my recovery. I remain healthy, happy, and optimistic!

But this does not mean that I am a Pollyanna. It does mean that I turned my determination (my family calls it stubbornness—and my reaction is, as always, "whatever!") into a focus (okay, obsession) with finding out everything I could about the relationship between diet and disease. And this research has resulted in a wealth of information on the relationship between food and health.

Think twice before you reach for that can of soda, or sugary fruit drink, or that ginormous bag of chips. Think about the heavy desserts and greasy fried foods drenched in unhealthy oils. Think about how you feel afterwards and take notice of how it affects your mood; you may choose not to eat or drink it then.

What we feed our bodies matters. If we don't feed and nourish it properly, it will make you sick and you may lose your mind—literally! Think about it!

Always encourage healthy decisions.
Surround yourself with positive people.
Think about the choices of foods you put in your body.
Exercise daily.
Maintain a healthy weight.
Get 7 to 8 hours of sleep daily.
Manage stress.
Meditate.
Give back.
Give thanks.

Love, Cristina

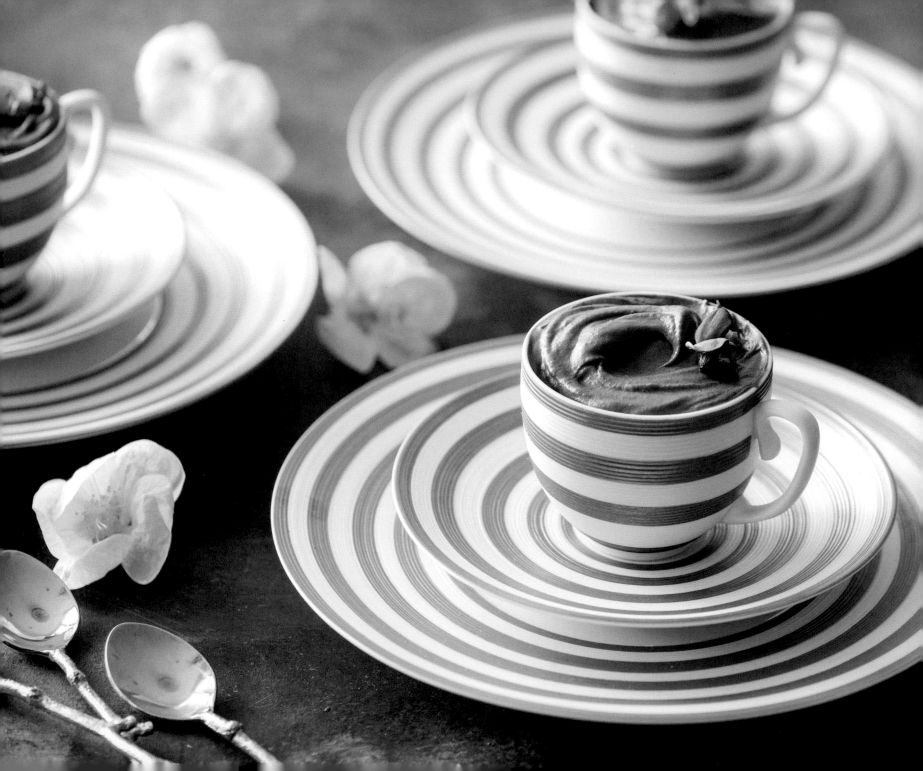

I just finished suggesting to you to eliminate processed sugar and dairy from your diet. Yes, this is a "Chocolate Mousse" for dessert, but it's made with no processed sugar, no dairy—no kidding! Look for it in the dessert section!

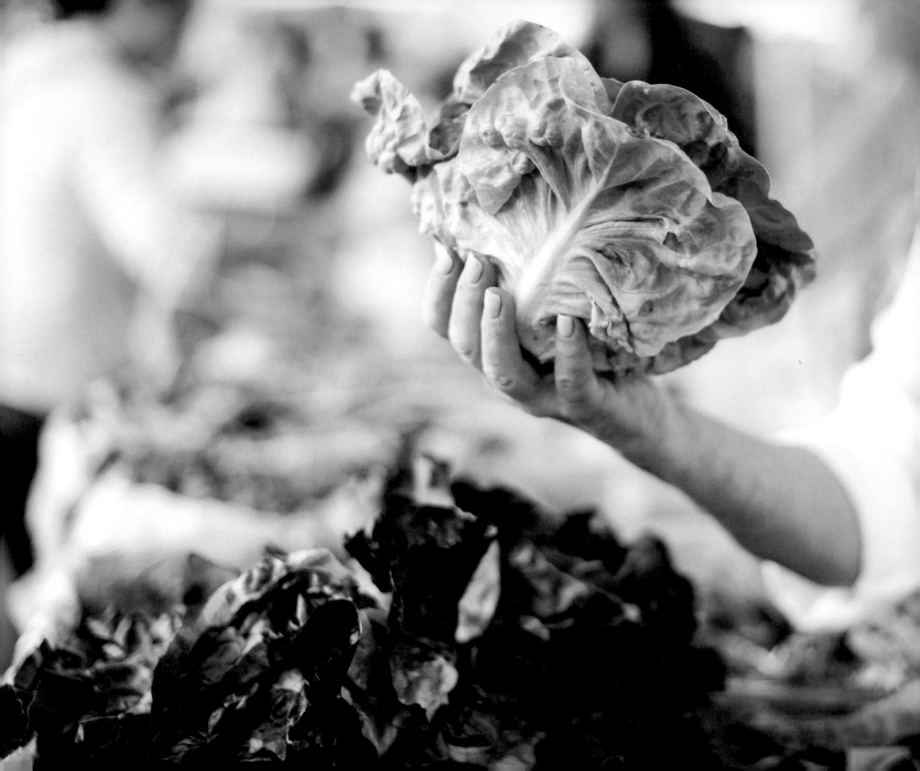

CHAPTER 1

Healing Foods

Do you ever stop to think, when you are about to bite into any piece of fruit, or eat a salad, or enjoy a bowl of soup, or eat anything, about the kinds of vitamins or nutrients you are giving your body? My guess would be no; I don't. Who does? But I want you to know that every ingredient I use in this book has a nutritional purpose. I want to share some of these ingredients and their benefits with you so you can feel good about what you're eating!

The Importance of Fruit in Your Diet

APPLE

Ever wonder why an apple a day keeps the doctor away? It's probably because apples are packed with nutritional benefits for the body and the brain. Adding an apple into your daily diet helps keep your brain healthy because of this fruit's high levels of the flavonoid *quercetin*. Quercetin is an antioxidant that helps prevent oxidation and inflammation in your brain's neurons, which can lead to cellular death. Reducing cellular death in the brain helps defend against the onset of dementia and Alzheimer's. Post-menopausal women should add apples into their diet to protect against osteoporosis and increase bone density.

BANANA

Americans consume more bananas than apples and oranges combined, so it shouldn't be hard to incorporate this healthy fruit into your diet. The banana is one of the best sources of potassium around. Potassium plays an important role in numerous functions in the body. It helps lower blood pressure because of its vasodilation effects, which means the widening of the blood vessels. When the blood vessels constrict, your blood pressure goes higher; when the blood vessels widen, your blood pressure lowers. Make sure to eat this popular fruit daily to maintain healthy potassium levels. Bananas also contain the chemical tryptophan that is also found in turkey. Tryptophan is a mood-enhancing chemical that can help you feel calmer and more relaxed.

BLUEBERRY

Blueberries are a sweet summer treat and a powerful brain food. Like raspberries and strawberries, blueberries contain anthocyanin, which is the compound that gives all these fruits their vibrant color. Anthocyanins are also powerful antioxidants that work wonders for brain health and can prevent neurological disorders like Parkinson's and Alzheimer's. Blueberries also contain another antioxidant called proanthocyanidins. The combination of the two antioxidants anthocyanin and proanthocyanidin pack a powerful punch for brain health because they stimulate mitochondria, brain cells' major energy source. Stimulation of the mitochondria helps your brain cells process energy more efficiently and ultimately helps alleviate neurodegeneration.

CANTALOUPE

This low-fat, high-flavor fruit is a great source of vitamin A, which is essential for eye health and helps promote healthy mucus membranes and skin. Cantaloupes are also a good source of potassium, which is necessary for cardiovascular health because it helps control blood pressure and heart rate. Maintaining healthy blood pressure and steady heart rate protects you against heart attacks and strokes. Looking to get a bunch of essential vitamins? Cantaloupes contain vitamin C, B-complex vitamins such as niacin, and manganese, which help support a healthy immune system, protect against free radicals, and work to remove toxins from the body. Cantaloupes also act as an anti-inflammatory because they are packed with phytonutrients that will prevent inflammation in the joints that can lead to arthritis.

CHERRY

Cherries are considered a superfood, which is a nutrient-rich food with numerous health benefits to the body. Indeed, these delicious fruits, especially the tart varieties, offer a powerful dose of antioxidants. Studies show that adding just one cup of tart cherries to your daily diet can help protect against arthritis, cancers, and cardiovascular issue. Cherries contain the antioxidant cyanidin, which protects against cancers and the deterioration of cells. The impressive anti-inflammatory properties in cherries are the key to prevention against arthritis and heart disease. Studies show that a diet high in cherries also helps to lower cholesterol.

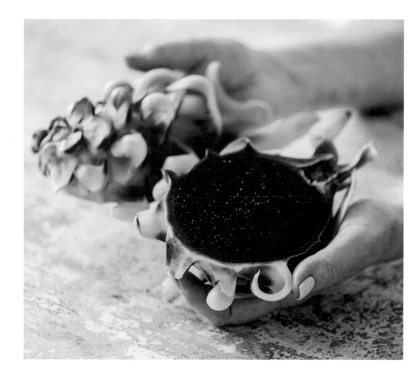

DRAGON FRUIT

Dragon fruit has a surprising number of phytonutrients and is rich in antioxidants. It also contains vitamin C equivalent to 10 percent of the daily value of polyunsaturated (good) fatty acids. Calcium is present for strong bones and teeth, iron and phosphorus for healthy blood and tissue formation. The benefits of dragon fruit are realized in a number of ways from a strengthened immune system and faster healing of bruises and wounds to fewer respiratory problems.

The seeds of dragon fruit are high in polyunsaturated fats (omega-3 and omega-6 fatty acids) that reduce triglycerides and lower the risk of cardiovascular disorders. Lycopene, responsible for the red color in dragon fruit, has been shown to be linked with a lower prostate cancer risk.

HONEYDEW

Honeydew melons are low in fat and are made up of about 90 percent water. Even though this refreshing fruit is mostly water, it is still filled with essential nutrients. Honeydews are a great source of potassium, which helps promote healthy blood pressure and heart rate. Getting the proper amount of potassium in your diet can also help prevent muscle cramps. One cup of cubed honeydew melon provides about 8 percent of your daily needed intake. Honeydews are also a great source of dietary fiber, which helps keep blood sugar low and steady. Fiber also helps keep digestion regular and prevents gastrointestinal disease. Another great source of vitamins, honeydews contain copper and B vitamins. Copper is an essential mineral for skin health because it helps regenerate skin cells. An insufficient intake of copper can also damage your body's ability to repair its muscles and tissues. Vitamin B is critical in helping your body rid itself of toxins that can cause illnesses like Alzheimer's.

LEMON

Lemons add freshness to many dishes and are a great finishing touch to a meal. This versatile fruit is packed with health benefits and high doses of essential vitamin C. Studies show that large amounts of citrus, including lemon, can help lower the risk of ischemic stroke in women. Ischemic strokes are caused by a blockage of the blood vessels in the brain. Additionally, lemons support overall brain health because they contain vitamin C and potassium, which help to support neurological wellness. The citric acid in lemons helps to dissolve calcium deposits, gallstones, and kidney stones in the body, so drinking lemon juice in your water may help prevent these painful disorders. Even your liver loves lemons because this tart fruit acts as both a liver detoxifier and stimulant.

LIME

Limes are in the same flavor family as lemons and have many of the same health benefits. Limes, like lemons, contain limonoids, a natural compound that helps fight cancerous cells. Limonoids stay in the body for a longer period of time than other antioxidants making them exceptionally bioavailable. The availability and persistence of limonoids is what makes them a beneficial compound to fight cancers. Limes are also especially good for post-menopausal and child-bearing women because of their high levels of folate and calcium, essential vitamins and minerals for women's health.

MANGO

Another great source of antioxidants, mangos contain the compound zeaxanthin, which assists with eye health by filtering out harmful blue rays that can cause macular degeneration. Mangos also contain beta-carotene. Studies show that diets high in vitamin A have fewer occurrences of cancers including colon, breast, and lung. Eating mangos is another way to lower "bad" LDL cholesterol because of the good dose of fiber and vitamin C found in this fruit. Also considered a fair source of iron, mango is a good choice to help you get closer to your daily iron intake, which is especially important to women.

PAPAYA

Like pineapple, papayas contain a unique digestive enzyme called papain that helps with the food digestion process. Papayas are heart healthy because they contain high levels of fiber and folic acid. Folic acid helps protect against the breakdown of blood vessel walls, which can cause a heart attack. Getting the proper amount of fiber in your diet can lower cholesterol. Papayas are also packed with high levels of vitamins C, vitamin A, and beta-carotene making this fruit a great choice to help support your immune system. Also, studies show that high doses of vitamin C help protect you against degenerative arthritic diseases like rheumatoid arthritis. Try incorporating papaya into your daily diet to increase your regular vitamin C intake.

PEACH

Besides being a delicious summer treat, peaches are filled with health benefits. In addition to high levels of vitamin C, stone fruits, like peaches, have particularly strong benefits for people who have diabetes and certain cancers. Peaches have high levels of fiber, which helps to slow the absorption of glucose into the blood and is beneficial for regulating blood sugars for diabetics. Also, studies show that the phenols, or antioxidants, in peaches attack cancerous breast cells, but do not damage regular, healthy cells. Some studies even claim that the antioxidants in peaches are superior to the ones found in blueberries.

PINEAPPLE

Pineapples are the only source of an enzyme called bromelain, a proteolytic enzyme, which helps break down proteins in the stomach. This important enzyme is anti-inflammatory and will aid in digestion. Eating pineapple for dessert after a heavy dinner will help your body process the meal faster by breaking down the contents of your stomach. Pineapple supports healthy, strong bones because of its high levels of the vitamin manganese. One cup of pineapple juice gives you about 73 percent of your required manganese intake for the day.

RASPBERRY

Like all of the other berries, raspberries are filled with antioxidants and polyphenols such as anthocyanins and flavonoids. This rich source of antioxidants can protect against the oxidative stress caused by free radicals. Each of these antioxidant compounds helps assist with different areas of the body. For example, flavonoids contribute to brain health and the effects of cognitive aging. Anthocyanins help reduce platelet build-up in the blood that can lead to cardiovascular disease. Also, these anthocyanins promote overall anti-inflammatory benefits to the body.

STRAWBERRY

These large berries are one of the best sources of antioxidants you can add to your diet. Strawberries contain a family of antioxidants called anthocyanins, which are the compounds that give the strawberry its rich red color. These anthocyanins have been widely studied for their effects on brain health and memory. The brain is made up almost entirely of fat. When fat begins to diminish in a brain, a person starts to experience memory and motor-function loss. Studies show that when a person receives high levels of anthocyanins, the brain will stop losing the fat it needs to thrive. Eating strawberries supports healthy fats in your brain. It is one of the best fat-burning foods for fast and easy weight loss.

WATERMELON

Summertime barbecues come to mind with this delicious fruit. Some people may think that watermelons are not nutritious because they are so sweet, but watermelons are indeed nutrient rich. Watermelons contain the antioxidant lycopene, which helps protect against the formation of free radicals that can cause heart disease and certain cancers. Also, watermelons have a high fiber content, which promotes healthy digestion and slows the absorption of sugars into the bloodstream. Watermelons may be eaten so frequently during the summer because they are made up of 92 percent water and essential electrolytes, so this fruit will help you stay hydrated during hot days. But this "summer treat" is a nutrient-rich snack to enjoy all year-round.

Health Benefits of Cooking Oils

COCONUT OIL

Coconut oil has become one of the more popular cooking oils in recent years. In the past, coconut oil has been overlooked as a healthy oil because of its high levels of saturated fats. Studies now show that saturated fats are not as detrimental to health as they were once believed, so coconut oil has moved to the forefront as one of the healthiest oils available. Some of the health benefits of coconut oil include fighting off bacteria and yeast, lowering cholesterol, and helping combat neurological diseases like Alzheimer's. Great for cardiovascular health, coconut oil contains the saturated fat lauric acid, which helps to increase "good" HDL cholesterol. Also, coconut oil promotes healthy thyroid function, which keeps cholesterol healthy. This is because when the thyroid is not working properly, your levels of bad cholesterol rise. Correct thyroid function has a direct correlation with healthy brain development.

Coconut oil holds many benefits for the brain. The brain needs healthy fats to thrive, and coconut oil provides nutritious fats that keep the brain from becoming toxic.

EXTRA-VIRGIN OLIVE OIL

This popular cooking oil is a great source of heart-healthy fats. In fact, olive oil is the main fat source for the Mediterranean diet, which is one of the healthiest diets around and statistically shows lower risk of heart disease and stroke for people from that region. This healthy fat source is made up mainly of monounsaturated fats, which can help lower "bad" LDL cholesterol, not contribute to it. Olive oil is also helpful in preventing cancers because of its high levels of polyphenol antioxidants, which prevent oxidative stress on your organs. These same polyphenol compounds have also been studied to reduce the risk of Alzheimer's disease. This is because polyphenols reduce oxidation in the brain that can lead to neurotoxicity, and olive oil contains certain polyphenols that are particularity powerful for the brain. People from the region who consume the Mediterranean diet have statistically fewer occurrences of diseases like Alzheimer's within their population.

GHEE

Ghee is similar to clarified butter, which is made by heating butter to remove the water and milk solids. When comparing ghee to butter, ghee is simmered longer which will bring out the butter's nutlike flavor. What I like about ghee is that it has a higher smoke point than butter. Ghee can be heated to a higher temperature before it starts to smoke. Most cooking oils with a high smoke point, such as canola, peanut, corn, and soybean oils, are usually genetically modified and often partially hydrogenated. Heating a cooking fat above its smoke point breaks down important phytonutrients and causes the fat to oxidize and form harmful free radicals.

Ghee is packed with fat-soluble vitamins that can be especially crucial if you suffer from any conditions like leaky gut syndrome, IBS, or Crohn's. Almost all supermarkets carry ghee. In recent years, ghee and clarified butter have gained popularity across the United States for their potential health benefits. Ghee is rich in vitamin A and vitamin E, and it is lactose-free.

GRAPESEED OIL

Grapeseed oil offers myriad health benefits. This nutritious oil contains linoleic acid, which has been studied as a way to reduce complications associated with diabetes, especially for the visual problems caused by this disease. Grapeseed oil can also repair broken and damaged capillaries and improve circulation. Poor blood circulation can lead to conditions like varicose veins, spider veins, and hemorrhoids. Another great source of antioxidants, grapeseed oil protects against colon, stomach, and breast cancers. Grapeseed oil also has applications in beauty and has been shown to relieve acne and dermatitis.

SESAME OIL

Sesame oil is another example of a delicious, heart-healthy oil. Full of mono- and polyunsaturated fats, sesame oil offers these nutritious fats that help cut down on cholesterol. Sesame oil also contains the unique antioxidants sesamol and sesamin, which protect against cardiovascular disease and cancers. Applying sesame oil directly to the skin has even been studied to help reduce the risk of skin cancers like melanoma. This oil also packs a good dose of fiber, so drizzle it on your salad to get closer to your daily fiber intake, also important for digestive health. It is is a good choice for diabetics; studies show that ingesting sesame oil regularly helps decrease blood sugar levels and increase antioxidants in the blood.

WALNUT OIL

Walnut oil is a great source of healthy monounsaturated fats such as omega-9, which helps keep arteries flexible. Supple arteries promote blood flow, which helps prevent hypertension and heart disease. Omega fatty acids found in walnut oil also reduce inflammation that can lead to diseases like arthritis. Incorporating walnut oil into your diet can also help regulate proper hormone levels. Minerals found in walnut oil, like zinc, iron, and calcium, are great at stabilizing hormones in your body. Studies show that ingesting walnut oil can even help prevent certain cancers because it contains high levels of ellagic acid. Ellagic acid has been shown to kill cancer cells and break down carcinogens in the liver.

The Dangers of Processed Sugar

The medical definition of a poison is: "Any substance applied to the body, ingested or developed within the body, which causes or may cause disease." When sugars are refined, they are depleted of any nutritional value including vitamins and minerals. All that is left is refined starch and carbohydrate, which the body is unable to utilize. Added vitamins and minerals in a substance allow the body to metabolize, or properly digest, carbohydrates. Without these essential vitamins and minerals, carbohydrates metabolize into a toxic substance that acts as a poison to the body. During the metabolization process, sugars leach vitamins and minerals from the body as the carbohydrates try to properly digest. Eating sugars actually removes positive nutrients from your body and leaves toxicity.

A recent study published in the Journal of the International Neuropsychological Society suggests exercise can build up a part of your brain that withers with Alzheimer's disease. Researchers at the University of Maryland School of Public Health put older adults on a moderate-intensity exercise program and found that the thickness of the outer layer of the brain—called the cortex—increased, potentially offering protection against dementia.

So how much exercise do you need? In a study published recently in the Journal of Alzheimer's Research, researchers found that 150 minutes of moderate exercise per week—the CDC's recommendation for adults—can significantly improve memory performance after just 12 weeks.

Important Food Types

HERBS

When you are trying to use less fat and salt in your diet, using fresh herbs adds so much flavor that you will find yourself not reaching for the salt shaker or missing the flavor of heavy fats. Not only do fresh herbs enhance your recipes, but they are also filled with super health benefits. I add fresh herbs to most everything I make.

Looking to add extra flavor and nutrition to your recipes? Fresh herbs are the answer. Herbs are packed with vitamins and nutrients that can easily be incorporated into your daily diet.

Studies on using fresh herbs in your diet have shown a reduction in cardiovascular disease, increase in positive brain health, and anti-inflammatory properties. Additionally, herbs can act as a great flavor alternative to heavy fats like butter and salts. Substituting herbs for fats or sodium to pump up flavor will make your dish lower in calories and more nutrient rich.

Diets containing a range of fresh herbs and are low in fats can be most successful. The Mediterranean diet, for example, uses many of the herbs used in my recipes. Studies show that people who eat a Mediterranean diet have fewer occurrences of obesity, heart disease, and neurological disorders like Alzheimer's and Parkinson's.

Make sure to incorporate as many fresh herbs and spices as you can into your diet, as they contain many health benefits. Basil, mint, rosemary, oregano, thyme, cilantro, parsley, chives, dill, sage, tarragon, bay leaf, sorrel, turmeric, cinnamon, mint, sage, and peppermint, to name a few, all have powerful anti-inflammatory effects on brain function and memory.

NUTS

Looking for a quick and healthy snack? Think about nuts, these tiny nutritional powerhouses are packed with protein, fiber, and various minerals. People who eat nuts as part of a daily diet can lower bad cholesterol in the blood and even reduce the risk of blood clots. A small portion of about 30 grams can both fill you up with healthy essential fats and provide important vitamins for your body.

I make sure to include in my diet every day, two times a day, a handful of walnuts, almonds, cashews, pistachios, chestnuts, macadamia nuts, pecans, or hazelnuts. I eat them as a snack, put them in salads and soups, and in my breakfast cereal, oatmeal, and yogurt!

LEGUMES

The hearty legume is an exceptional source of plant-based protein and can serve as a good alternative to high-fat protein sources like red meats. In fact, vegetarians look to beans as one of their main sources of protein. Beans are highly nutritious and are full of antioxidants, fiber, B vitamins, and key minerals, making them a valuable addition to anyone's diet.

Here is a list of my favorite beans: black beans, fava beans, butter beans, cannellini beans, Garbanzo Beans, edamame, great northern white beans, Italian beans, kidney beans, lima beans, navy beans, pinto beans, and white beans.

We have pesticides in our food, foods that are genetically modified, air that is toxic, treated water, chemicals in our body and laundry soaps, lotions, and shampoo, and everything comes to us wrapped in plastic. Plastic leaches even more toxins into our food and drink. Fast foods, sugary sodas, and desserts filled with even more sugar are being pumped into our bodies, every day, all day long, 365 days a year. Your body can only do so much to keep filtering out all these poisons. It's no wonder that eventually our minds and bodies are being chipped away, leaving a path for all kinds of cancer, heart disease, diabetes, and Alzheimer's.

Cookware

It's important to invest in really good cookware so I will start with what I think are the best pans to use for cooking. My preferences are stainless steel and cast iron. Make sure your pots and pans are stainless steel and not treated or coated aluminum because that will actually leach into the food as it cooks.

Professionals use copper pots but are very expensive and need to be maintained. They also react with acidic foods, such as changes in the flavor of a sauce as the copper reacts to the acid in tomatoes, for example.

Aluminum pans will leach chemicals into your food as it cooks. Cast-iron pots (my choice because they get really hot) are porous and grease can turn rancid if you don't season them properly. They must be completely dry so they don't rust, and seasoned with a coating of olive oil. Coated pans or Teflon will eventually chip off.

Stainless pots are great for cooking. They come in various thicknesses, so buy the best. Stainless steel by itself is not a good conductor of heat so look for pans with copper or aluminum cores. If you take proper care of them, they will last you a lifetime.

Stainless steel pots are extremely durable and will maintain their appearance for a very long time. I have pots handed down to me from my mom, and they are still the best pots ever! Stainless steel will not impart any flavor or create a chemical reaction with food.

Buy the best cookware. Make an investment in your health!

For those who are new to cooking, the first thing you need to know is this: You won't get anything to brown in nonstick coated cookware. Using stainless steel, copper, or cast-iron is the only way to get beautifully browned meats, but there are some important things to know about pans before you start cooking. Temperature is key, so learning to use your pots and pans is a good idea if you don't want to ruin your food and destroy your pots. If you don't know how to use them properly or how to manage the temperature, food will stick to the pan or burn.

Here are some important tips about cookware:

- Aluminum pans will actually leach aluminum into the food as it cooks.
- Copper pots are used by professionals but they are very expensive and difficult to maintain; they react with acidic foods.
- Glass pots have poor heat distribution and food will burn easily in them.
- Coated pans, no matter how expensive or well made, will eventually chip. What you don't see before the actual chipping begins are the minute particles that wear off and lead to chipping.
- The right types of utensils are needed for all types of pans, including stainless.

- Stainless is durable and can maintain its appearance for as long as you own it (some cooks who use stainless steel have had their cookware for as long as 50 years). Even the best stainless cookware will get tiny scratches if you use knives on them, but generally, stainless is resistant to scratches and dents.

Wash Your Fruits and Veggies

Wash your fruits and vegetables, especially if they are not organic, in a fruit and veggie wash. Fill a large bowl with 3 quarts of water and 1 cup plain white vinegar. Soak fruit or vegetables for 10 minutes. Rinse well with water, preferably filtered.

Appliances, Cookware, Utensils, and Pantry Staples

The best thing is that if you keep your pantry and refrigerator stocked with these items, you will ensure that you will always have a meal for your family or last-minute guests, always!

The following is an essential list of important appliances, cookware, utensils, and pantry staples you should have in your kitchen.

APPLIANCES

High-powered blender
Food processor
Juicer
Knife sharpener
Citrus squeezer

COOKWARE

3 cast-iron skillets: 1 large, 2 medium-sized
Cast-iron grill pan
Stainless steel pots: 4-quart soup pot,
    3-quart saucepot

UTENSILS

High-quality knives: chef's knife, serrated, paring, boning, utility, carving.

Set of metal tongs

Set of measuring cups and measuring spoons

Wooden spoons

Spatulas

Funnel

Pyrex liquid measuring cup

Kitchen scale

Chinois or China cap: A chinois (also called a China cap), is a cone-shaped metal strainer with a very fine mesh. It is used for straining stocks, sauces, soups, and other items that need to have a smooth consistency. (Highly recommended.)

Wooden cutting board

Set of plastic cutting boards: a color-coded set should include boards for vegetables, chicken, beef, fish, and fruit

Salad spinner

Bowls: stacked, glass, and stainless-steel

Carbon steel wok

Steamer, for vegetables

Mason jars, 12 quart-sized, 12 pint-sized

Mandoline (vegetable slicer)

Zester

Cheese grater

PANTRY STAPLES

Oils: extra-virgin olive oil, coconut oil

Fresh lemons (6)

Kosher salt

Boxed soups: organic vegetable, chicken, beef

Garlic

Yellow onions

Shallots (3)

Dijon mustard

2 (28-ounce) cans organic chopped tomatoes

2 (28-ounce) cans organic tomato purée

2 jars of your favorite pasta sauce

Pasta assortment

Canned beans: black, navy, cannelini, pinto, garbanzo

Canned Thai coconut milk

Canned coconut cream

Sriracha hot sauce

Lite soy sauce, gluten-free soy sauce (Tamari)

Regular or vegan mayonnaise

Monk fruit sweetener

Organic peanut butter

Assorted nuts and seeds: whole organic walnuts, almonds, pecans, hazelnuts, pumpkin seeds, sesame seeds, sunflower seeds

Unsweetened coconut or almond milk

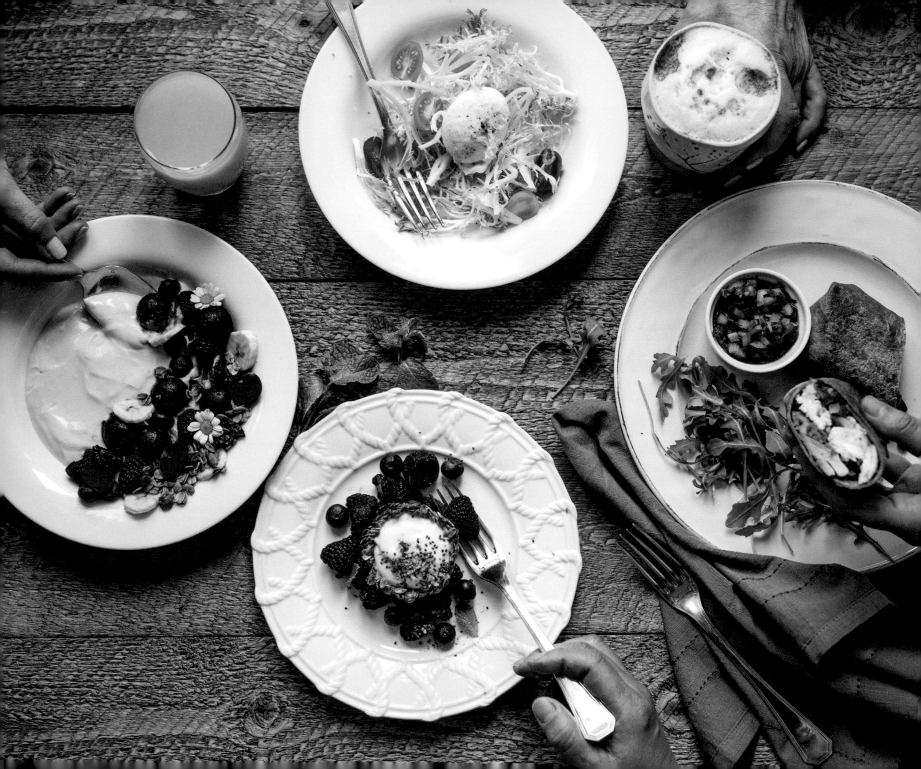

CHAPTER 2

Breakfast, Good Morning!

The Importance of Eating Breakfast

I love breakfast! Breakfast breaks the overnight fasting period after a night's sleep. Most of all, eating a healthy breakfast is important for overall health and weight management, it replenishes glucose and provides essential nutrients to keep your energy levels up throughout your day.

A good breakfast burns fat, helps keep blood sugar level, helps fight daytime cravings, keeps the brain sharp, and helps with concentration and productivity.

A nutritious breakfast will help energize your body, clear your mind, and keep you active and productive until lunch.

All these results are in every breakfast recipe in this chapter. (Unless you are having doughnuts, in which case we need to have an entirely different conversation!)

Protein jumpstarts your metabolism, makes you feel fuller longer, and helps avoid midmorning cravings.

Fiber from fruits, vegetables, and whole grains will help with digestion and deliver powerful antioxidants.

Breakfast is the most important meal of the day and has an abundance of sound science behind it. According to the Food Research and Action Center, "The correlation between breakfast and school performance among children based on numerous research findings include how eating and not eating breakfast affects academics, brain function, and overall wellness. Children who eat breakfast do better in school."

Make sure to offer a variety of different foods for breakfast, such as whole wheat or whole grain breakfast cereals, eggs, oats, organic fresh fruits, and yogurt.

Also offer breads such as whole wheat, multigrain, seeded whole grain, and whole wheat bagels.

Fresh fruit juices, smoothies, and nut milks, such as unsweetened almond milk, coconut milk, hazelnut milk, cashew milk, and organic low-fat milk, are nutritious. Take the time to eat breakfast—it will make a difference in your day!

I wanted to start the breakfast chapter by getting back to basics—eggs. Eggs seem to have lost their place in the breakfast world because people are still not sure if eggs are good for you. I assure you, they are.

Eggs are one of the most nutritious foods available and contain your daily needed intakes of these vitamins: vitamin A, 6 percent; folate, 5 percent; vitamin B_5, 7 percent; vitamin B_{12}, 9 percent; vitamin B_2, 15 percent; phosphorus, 9 percent; and selenium, 22 percent.

Eating one large egg is a great way to make sure you get these essential vitamins into your diet. Benefits from eating eggs can only be experienced when they form part of a balanced diet. They build strong muscles, are good for brain health and energy production, keep the immune system healthy, and help lower the risk of heart disease.

At least twice during the week, and always for Sunday brunch, I prepare eggs, and when I do, I want them to be perfect—or should I say, my family would like for them to be perfect. Over the years of hearing my eggs were too runny, too hard, too soft, jiggle too much, are not fluffy, or are too fluffy, I have perfected the egg to my family's liking. I spent a whole day in the kitchen to go over in detail the cooking times, techniques, and ingredients on how to prepare eggs. I went through several dozen eggs and my whole house smelled like sulphur, but it was worth it in the end.

Let's get started!

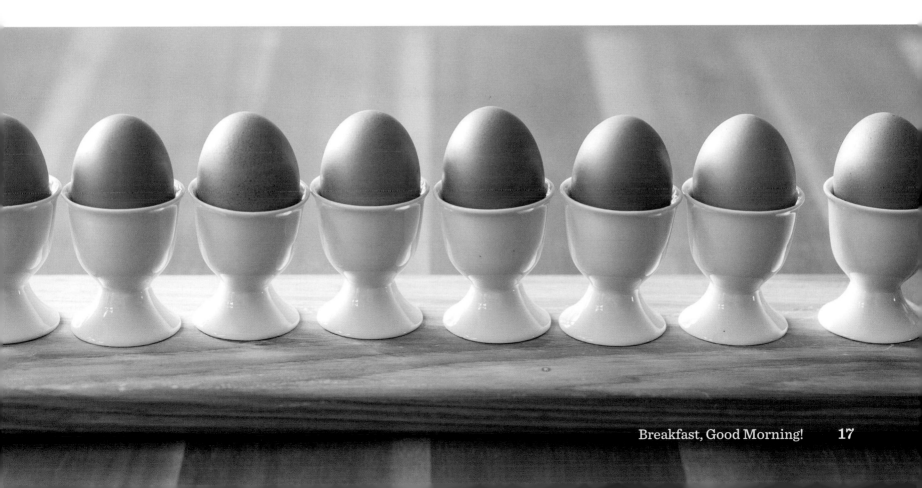

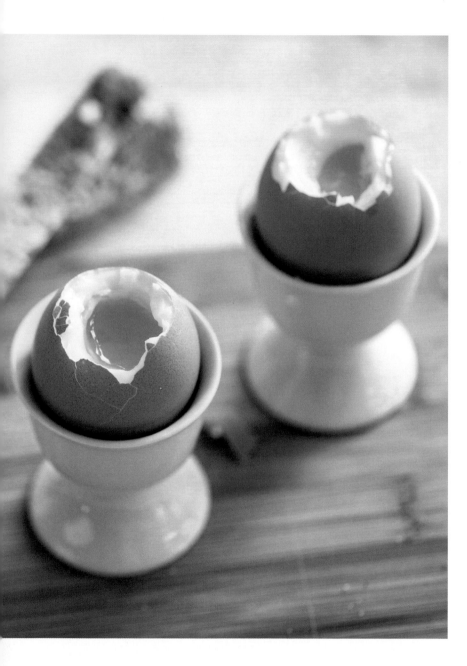

Soft Boiled Dip-in Eggs

SERVES 2

INGREDIENTS

2 slices multigrain or multi-seeded bread
4 large eggs
2 tablespoons coconut butter
Pinch of large coarse sea salt or truffle salt
Pinch of cracked black pepper

INSTRUCTIONS

1. Toast the bread, cover with a kitchen towel, and set aside.

2. Gently place the eggs into the bottom of a small-to medium-sized saucepan and cover with water, about 2 inches over the eggs.

3. Turn the heat to high and bring the eggs to a boil. Lower the heat and gently boil for 2½ minutes.

4. Remove the eggs from the boiling water using a slotted spoon and place them into a small bowl. Immediately run the eggs under cold water for 20 seconds to stop the eggs from cooking in their own heat.

5. Tap the top of each egg with a teaspoon to crack the shell and peel it down one inch. Use a teaspoon to lift the egg white to reveal the yolk and sprinkle it with a pinch of your favorite salt and pepper.

6. Spread the toast with coconut butter and cut into strips to dip into the creamy yolks! Enjoy!

Fluffy Scrambled Eggs

The secret to fluffy creamy scrambled eggs is patience; they need to cook low and slow. Salting eggs before they are scrambled tends to toughen them, so I salt my eggs after they are cooked with kosher salt or a flavored finishing salt.

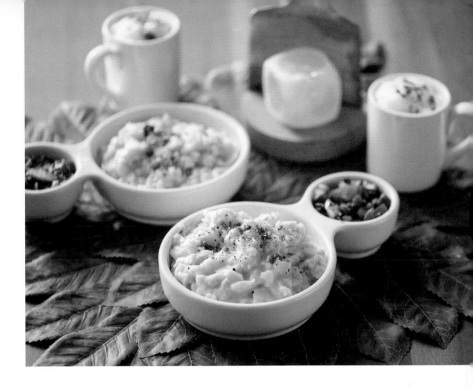

SERVES 4

INGREDIENTS

8 organic eggs

3 tablespoons 2% dairy or cashew milk

Organic coconut cooking spray

2 tablespoons organic whipped vegan spread cut into pieces

4 fresh basil leaves, rolled and thinly sliced into ribbons

2 teaspoons chopped chives

Kosher salt and cracked black pepper

Tomato slices, optional

Avocado slices, optional

INSTRUCTIONS

1. Crack the eggs into a medium-sized bowl and pierce the yolks with a fork. Add the milk and whisk until well combined.

2. Spray an 8-inch skillet generously with the coconut cooking spray. Add the eggs and the vegan spread.

3. Set the heat to medium and use chopsticks to constantly move the eggs back and forth, especially on the sides of the pan, until they start to set into small curds and look wct. If you don't have chopsticks, use a rubber spatula and scrape along the bottom and sides of skillet towards the middle to fluff the eggs. This will takc a fcw minutes as you want them to be light, smooth, and creamy.

4. If you prefer your eggs to be drier, continue to cook until they reach your desired level of doneness. Immediately transfer the eggs to a warm plate and garnish with the basil and chopped chives. Salt and pepper to taste.

5. I serve 2 slices of tomatoes and one-quarter of an avocado on the side with a drizzle of olive oil and a crunchy piece of toast or half of a hollowed bagel!

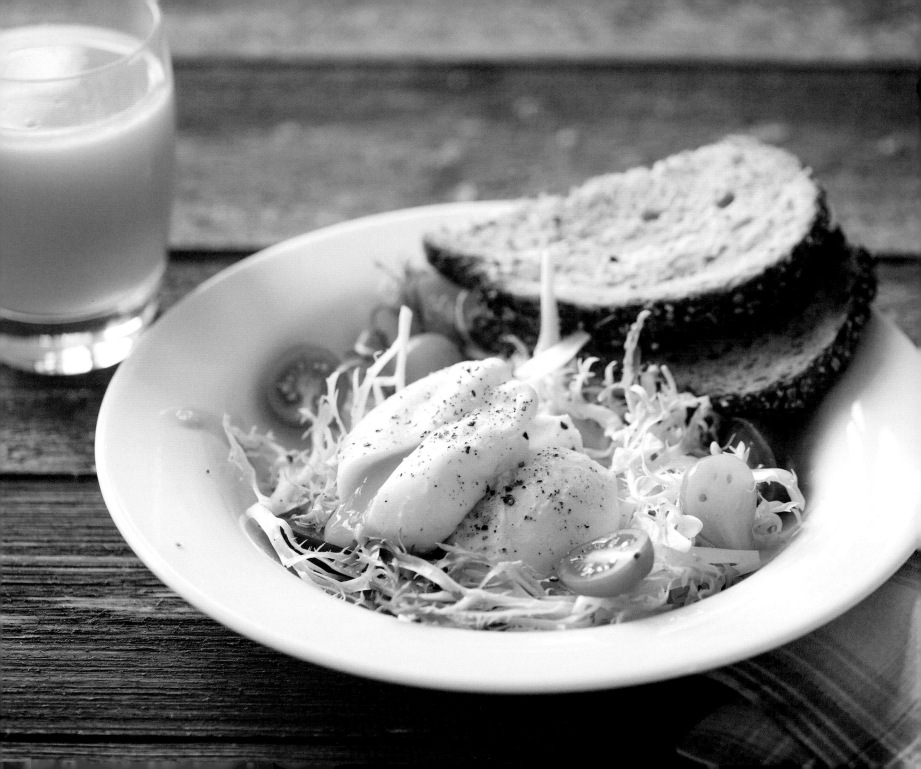

Perfectly Poached Eggs

When I first tried to poach eggs, I watched most of the egg whites float to the top of the water and congeal, looking like little fluffy floating islands, leaving the yolk at the bottom in a tiny ball all by itself. I researched every trick in the book to come up with a poached egg technique that has egg whites that surround and hold the creamy yolk in place. I finally achieved what I was looking for, and you can too, if you follow these easy steps.

SERVES 4

INGREDIENTS

2 tablespoons white wine vinegar

4 organic eggs

3 cups frisée lettuce

12 baby Roma tomatoes, sliced in half top to bottom, or cherry tomatoes, sliced in half

Kosher salt

Olive oil

INSTRUCTIONS

1. Fold 3 paper towels to double thickness and lay them on the counter next to the stove.

2. Fill a medium-sized saucepan with 1 quart of water, add the vinegar, and bring to a gentle rolling boil.

3. Break each egg separately into a custard cup. Quickly slip the first egg into the water, adding the rest of the eggs the same way. Poach 2 minutes per egg.

4. Remove the eggs (starting with the first one) with a slotted spoon and gently place it onto one of the folded paper towels to absorb excess water. Remove the others and serve immediately.

5. Serve with a handful of the frisée, tomatoes, a pinch of salt, a drizzle of olive oil, and your favorite seeded or whole wheat toast. or whole wheat bagel.

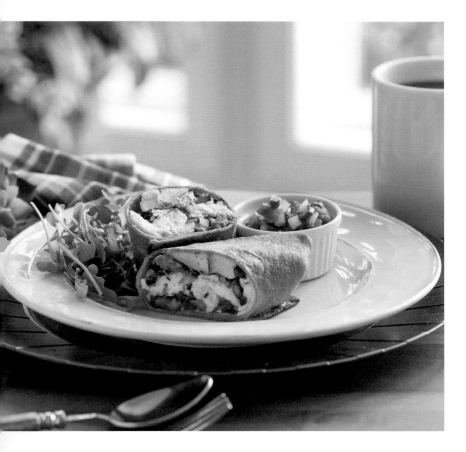

Egg White Protein Wrap

SERVES 4

INGREDIENTS

1 large ripe avocado at room temperature, peeled, pitted, and quartered

1 tablespoon fresh lemon juice

Organic coconut cooking spray

4 (10-inch) whole wheat or corn tortillas (also available gluten free)

10 egg whites

¼ cup coconut milk

¼ teaspoon each kosher salt

¼ teaspoon cracked black pepper

1½ cups shredded extra-sharp white cheddar cheese

2 cups black beans, drained and rinsed

2 jalapeños, seeded and sliced thin, optional

¾ cup Tomato Salsa, store-bought or homemade (see recipe, p. 217), plus more for serving

2 cups baby arugula

6 sprigs cilantro, leaves coarsely chopped (discard stems)

INSTRUCTIONS

1. Preheat the oven to 200F°.

2. Sprinkle the lemon juice over the avocado; cover and set aside.

3. Spray a 10- to 12-inch skillet lightly with cooking spray. Heat the skillet on medium for 1 minute. Place 1 tortilla in the skillet for 30 to 45 seconds. Turn it over and cook the other side.

4. Wrap tortillas in a kitchen towel and place them in the oven on a baking sheet. Keep all the tortillas wrapped and warmed in the oven until you are ready to serve.

5. In a medium mixing bowl, whisk the egg whites and coconut milk.

6. Spray the skillet you used for the tortillas with cooking spray. Turn the heat to medium and pour in the egg mixture. Using a wooden spoon, constantly stir and fluff the egg whites until they are cooked through, about 2 to 3 minutes. Season with salt and pepper.

7. Remove the skillet from heat and sprinkle the cheddar cheese evenly over the cooked egg mixture; cover with a lid and let sit for 2 minutes, or until the cheese has melted.

TO ASSEMBLE

1. On a chopping board, lay out the tortillas one at a time. Make sure you leave a space of 1½ inches open all around the tortilla to make it easier to roll and tuck them.

2. Mash the avocado lightly with a fork. Spread ¼ of the avocado on the lower third of a tortilla, and top with ¼ cup of the black beans and several jalapeños, if desired.

3. Divide the cooked egg whites equally into fourths. Place a quarter of the egg whites over the beans, followed by 2 tablespoons of salsa, ½ cup of baby arugula, and the cilantro.

4. Take the bottom of each tortilla and snuggly roll it over the filling, tucking in each side of tortilla; continue to roll it up tightly.

5. Spray coconut oil in a clean skillet and place the rolled tortillas inside with the seam side down.

6. On medium high heat lightly brown the outside of the tortilla on all sides. Remove from the skillet, slice in half, and serve with extra salsa on the side.

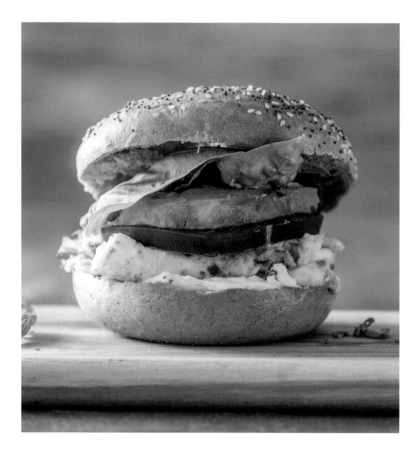

Hollowed Out Breakfast Bagel with Egg Whites and Herbed Cream Cheese

SERVES 2

INGREDIENTS

4 ounces low-fat cream cheese, room temperature

1 tablespoon chives, finely chopped

2 scallions, white and light green parts only, finely chopped

2 teaspoons finely chopped jalapeño

2 tablespoons extra-virgin olive oil

½ red bell pepper, seeded, chopped small

Coconut cooking spray

6 egg whites

¼ teaspoon kosher salt, plus more for seasoning

2 whole wheat seeded bagels, split in half, hollowed out, and toasted

1 avocado, peeled, pitted, and sliced (see Tip)

2 ¼-inch-thick slices organic tomato

8 fresh basil leaves

INSTRUCTIONS

1. In a small bowl combine the cream cheese, chives, scallions, and jalapeño. Mix until all ingredients are incorporated and the mixture is smooth.

2. In an 8-inch skillet on medium heat, add the olive oil and heat for 30 seconds. Add the bell pepper; sauté 2 minutes. Place into a small bowl and set aside.

3. Wipe the skillet down and spray it generously with coconut cooking spray.

4. Whisk the egg whites until foamy, about 30 seconds. Add the bell peppers and ¼ teaspoon salt; whisk until combined.

5. Heat the skillet on medium heat for 30 seconds. Add the egg whites and cook 2 minutes. Gently flip them over using a metal spatula; cook 2 more minutes.

6. Remove the egg whites from the heat and slice in half down the middle. Take each half and fold in half from top to bottom.

TO ASSEMBLE

For each sandwich, spread 2 generous tablespoons of the cream cheese mixture on the bottom half of the bagel, all the way around. Add half of the folded egg white, half of the avocado, 1 tomato slice, a pinch of salt, and 4 basil leaves. Add the bagel top.

Tip: Squeeze lemon juice over the avocado slices to keep them from turning brown.

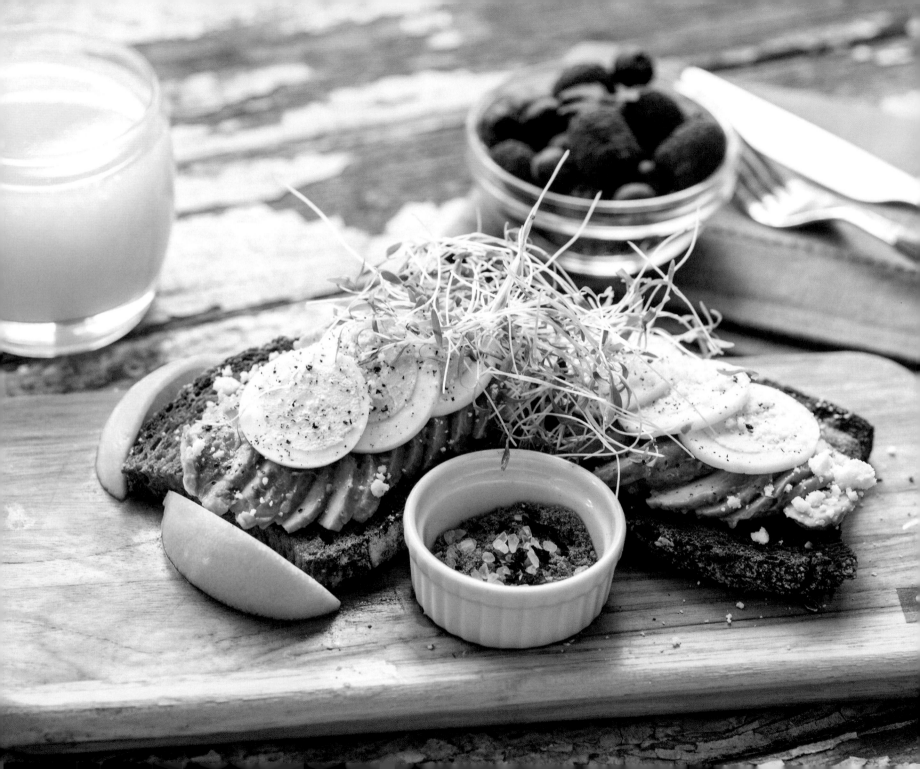

Avocado Toast

I eat a small avocado every day; I am addicted to them. I eat avocados plain with a squeeze of lemon juice and a pinch of salt, just because. I toss them into just about all my salads, use them in soups (I even have a recipe for an avocado soup in the Soups chapter that is one of my all-time favorites), put them in smoothies, garnish most dishes with them, and, of course, everyone's favorite, I make a mean guacamole! It is a "good morning" for me whenever I start my day with one of my favorite breakfasts, Avocado Toast.

Avocados are important for your memory! Some people may shy away from avocados because they think they are high in fat. The truth, however, is that avocados contain healthy fats and vitamins that are highly beneficial to the body and the brain. The brain is about 60 percent fat, and it needs nutritious fats like those found in avocados to function properly. The good fats and fiber in avocados can naturally help lower LDL and raise your "good" HDL cholesterol, help regulate blood sugar, and helps to alleviate inflammation throughout the body and brain.

Avocados are considered as one of the healthiest foods in the world. They contain over 25 essential vitamins and minerals, including vitamins A, B, C, E, and K, copper, iron, magnesium, and potassium.

SERVES 2

INGREDIENTS

4 slices whole wheat multigrain seeded bread, or an olive bread sliced into ½-inch-thick pieces, toasted

2 tablespoons ground cumin

½ teaspoon sea salt

⅛ teaspoon cayenne pepper

2 ripe avocados, peeled, pitted, and cut lengthwise into ¼-inch-thick slices

2 tablespoons crumbled feta cheese

1 cup microgreens, rinsed well; pat dry with a paper towel

Cracked black pepper to taste

2 lemon wedges

2 large eggs, boiled or poached

INSTRUCTIONS

1. In a small bowl combine the cumin, salt, and cayenne pepper. Mix well.

2. On each piece of toast place an avocado half. Gently fan out the avocado slices across the toast. Sprinkle ½ teaspoon of the cumin and salt mixture and 1 tablespoon feta cheese; top with a handful of the microgreens. Season with pepper and add a lemon wedge on the side.

3. Bring the cumin salt to the table as you will probably want to sprinkle more on!

4. I like to include a protein, so I add a boiled or poached egg over the top! Enjoy!

Tip: Squeeze 1 tablespoon of lemon juice over the avocado slices to prevent them from turning brown.

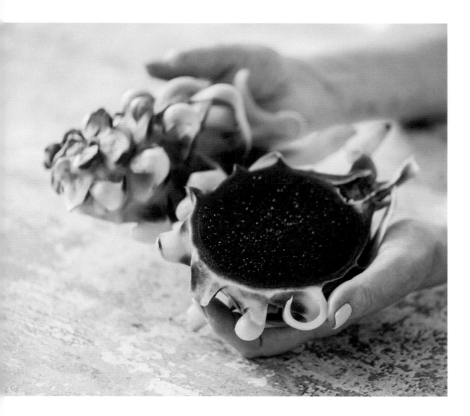

Dragons, Flowers, and Yogurt

This recipe calls for dragon fruit. If you can't find them you can use any melon you like.

If you have never heard of or used dragon fruit, here are some of the reasons why your health will benefit from adding this beautiful and colorful fruit in your diet.

Dragon fruit has many health benefits. It will help lower cholesterol, boost energy, strengthen the immune system, and improve digestion. Dragon fruit are rich in antioxidants and contain vitamins B and C. It is a rich source of calcium and iron and is high in omega-3 and omega-6 fatty acids.

The seeds will act as a mild laxative. Just thought I would throw that in there.

Yogurt has strains of "good bacteria" that are found in many yogurt products. Research is still being conducted on the many health benefits of yogurt in your diet. There is evidence that some strains of probiotics can boost the immune system and promote a healthy digestive tract. Yogurt contains calcium, protein, potassium, and other nutrients for maintaining bone health. These nutrients help prevent osteoporosis, which is a weakening of the bones.

SERVES 2

INGREDIENTS

2 cups Greek yogurt

Natural blue food color
(available online or at most markets)

1 dragon fruit (or your favorite melon),
cut into 10 to 12 balls

12 fresh raspberries

12 fresh blackberries

10 fresh blueberries

1 small banana, sliced

4 tablespoons of your favorite granola

1 teaspoon chia seeds

Edible flowers (available online)

4 fresh mint leaves

2 teaspoons of organic honey (optional)

INSTRUCTIONS

1. To color the yogurt, place it into a small bowl, add one or two drops of blue food color, and mix.

2. Spread 1 cup of the yogurt into each of the bottoms of two bowls.

3. Divide the dragon fruit or melon, raspberries, blackberries, blueberries, banana, granola, chia seeds, edible flowers, and mint evenly into the bowls.

4. Drizzle 1 teaspoon of organic honey over the top of each, if desired.

5. Have fun decorating the bowl anyway you like!

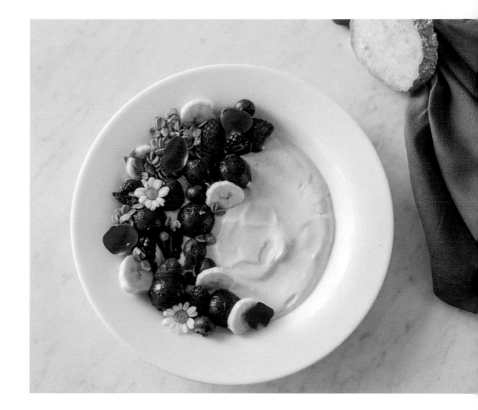

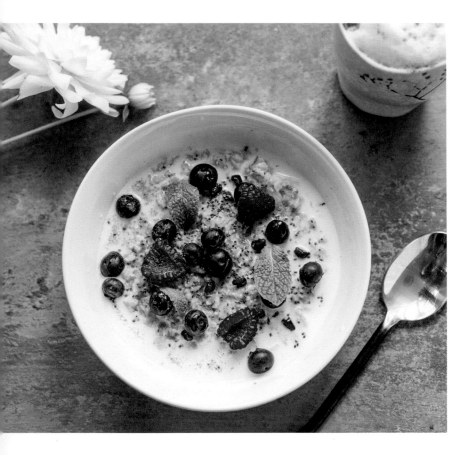

Old-Fashioned Oats for a New Way of Thinking

I eat a bowl of oatmeal with fresh blueberries, raspberries, and dragon fruit (when I can get it) at least three times a week. I add ground cinnamon to my oatmeal because of its anti-inflammatory properties. I need to keep my cholesterol in check and eating oats has been instrumental in helping me lower my LDL (bad cholesterol).

Studies have shown that oats are considered one of the healthiest grains and contain many health benefits. Oats are gluten free, high in fiber and protein, lower blood sugar, lower cholesterol levels, and help reduce the risk of heart disease.

One of the benefits of consuming oats is their effect on your blood cholesterol levels. Although you need some cholesterol in your bloodstream to help maintain your body's hormone balance, elevated cholesterol levels increase the risk of cardiovascular disease. The soluble fiber found in oats binds to cholesterol molecules in your intestinal tract, preventing those molecules from entering your bloodstream. I think that is amazing!

SERVES 2

INGREDIENTS

1½ cups water

⅛ teaspoon salt

8 raisins or dried cranberries, optional

1 cup rolled oats

1 cup dairy milk or your favorite nut milk (such as almond, hazelnut, cashew, or coconut milk)

¼ teaspoon ground cinnamon

½ teaspoon chia seeds

½ teaspoon hemp seeds

2 tablespoons pure maple syrup, divided between 2 servings

¼ cup fresh raspberries or blueberries, or a combination!

INSTRUCTIONS

1. Prepare 2 bowls by adding hot water to the bowls and letting them sit to take the chill off.

2. Bring the water, salt, and raisins or dried cranberries to a gentle boil in a small saucepan. Reduce the heat to medium-low, sprinkle in the oatmeal, and stir. Cook 4 minutes. Remove the pan from heat, cover with a lid, and let stand 3 minutes.

3. In another small saucepan, heat the milk or nut milk until small bubbles form on the side of the pan. The milk will be hot but not boiling.

4. Divide the oatmeal between the two preheated bowls. For each serving sprinkle the cinnamon, chia seeds, hemp seeds, and 1 tablespoon each of the maple syrup if desired. Add your choice of the warmed milk and the fresh berries.

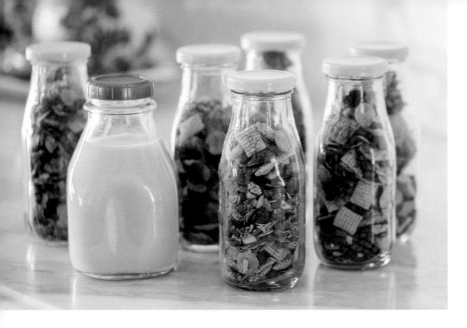

Make Your Own Cereal Mix

Some mornings I find myself in such a hurry to get out the door that don't have the time to make eggs, a smoothie, a yogurt bowl, or even wait for toast to get crispy. But I truly believe that starting your day off on a positive note by eating breakfast is important to fuel your brain and body and sustain you through the morning.

You can make your favorite combination of organic, sugar-free, and gluten-free cereal mix instead of opening up a box of sugary or empty calorie cereal. Here is what you can do in a hurry that will fuel you and your kids.

This recipe is a combination of my personal favorite cereals that I chose for my mix. Your kids can make their own cereal combination, and they will more likely go for it because they made it themselves!

MAKES 10 CUPS (1½ POUNDS)

INGREDIENTS

2 cups shredded wheat

1 cup of your favorite Kasha cereal

3 cups puffed rice cereal

3 cups organic wheat flakes

2 tablespoons ground cinnamon

2 teaspoons ground nutmeg

1 cup dried cherries

1 cup raisins

½ cup pumpkin seeds

2 tablespoons hemp seeds

2 tablespoons chia seeds

Your favorite dairy milk or nut milk, for serving

INSTRUCTIONS

1. Place all ingredients in a large bowl and mix well using your hands. Place the cereal mixture into 8 individual single-serving glass bottles (which are available at craft stores), or any other containers, such as glass Mason jars.

2. Place the leftover cereal in a Mason jar and store in the pantry until you need to fill up the bottles again!

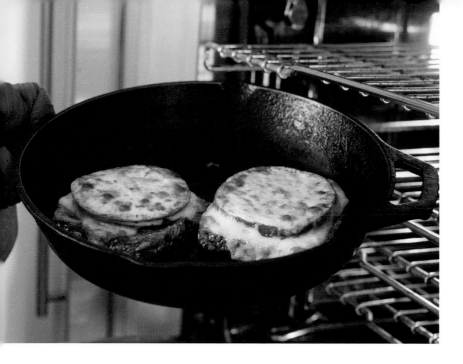

Cheesy Toast

Everyone in our family loves cheesy toast for breakfast! It's like having a grilled cheese sandwich but without all that butter, extra cheese, and extra bread that we don't really need to eat, especially in the morning.

This easy dish can be prepared quickly. It's light yet satisfying and won't sit in your tummy promising to cause problems later. I make this for lunch too, and I'll serve it with a bowl of soup or a light salad. I often follow it up with a steamy latte. Ahhh.

SERVES 4

INGREDIENTS

4 slices dense multigrain or multi-seeded bread, toasted

4 tablespoons Dijon mustard

4 medium organic Heirloom tomatoes, sliced ½-inch-thick

Organic Kosher salt and cracked black pepper, to taste

4 slices extra-thick, extra-sharp Vermont white cheddar cheese (see Cook's Note)

1 cup microgreens (available at most food markets)

INSTRUCTIONS

1. Place the oven rack 4 inches from the heat source and set the broiler to high.

2. Place the toasted bread in an ovenproof skillet (my preference is always a cast-iron skillet).

3. Spread one tablespoon of the Dijon over each slice of toast. Top with a tomato slice and sprinkle a pinch of salt and pepper over the top.

4. Lay one slice of the cheddar cheese over the tomato. Place the ovenproof dish under the broiler to melt the cheese. It won't take long, so *don't walk away*.

5. Remove the cheesy toast when the cheese has completely melted and starts to bubble and gets a bit crusty.

6. Serve with a steamy, hot latte or herbal tea!

Cook's Note: If you can't find extra-thick slices of Cheddar cheese in your deli sections just use two regular slices for each serving.

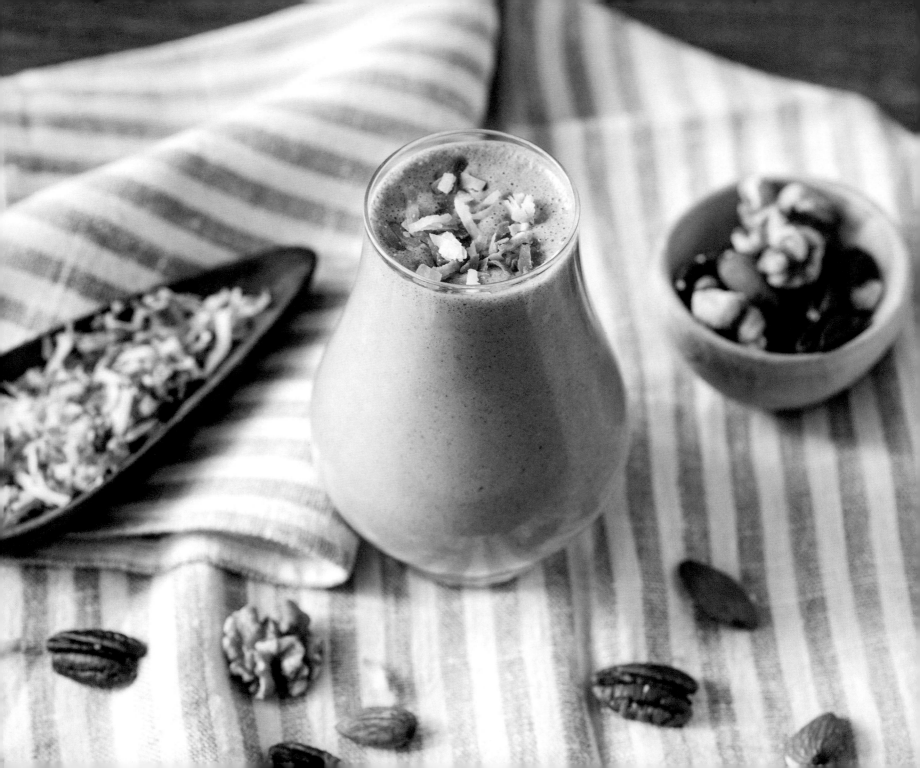

CHAPTER 3

Anytime Smoothies

There are many important reasons to incorporate smoothies into your daily diet. Not only are they delicious, they are filled with vital nutrients, minerals, vitamins, and antioxidants to help keep your brain, hcart, gut, and whole body strong. The many fruits and vegetables included in my smoothies are filled with phytonutrients and are rich in vitamins and minerals.

I use pineapple, papaya, coconut, pomegranates, and mangos. These fruits are a great source of vitamin C, potassium, folate, and manganese, which keep your bones, blood sugar, thyroid, and nerves healthy and your mind sharp. Peaches, citrus, berries, cherries, melons, apples, bananas, and pears provide beta-carotene and potassium, which help vision and help the immune system to function properly.

One serving of these fruits typically contains two to four grams of fiber with blackberries, pears, and apples having the highest concentration. All of the smoothies in this chapter are enhanced even further by the addition of more nutrients that come from nut milks, nuts, herbs, flax seed, chia seeds, hemp, and cacao.

When my kids were in school, I would always have a smoothie ready for them afterward to boost their energy levels and help prevent "homework meltdown." It also gave me time to sit down and ask about their day. Sometimes I'd make the smoothies in the morning and store them in the refrigerator so they would be ready later.

Even though consuming fruit is important to your health by supplying essential vitamins and minerals, our bodies convert these naturally into forms of sugar for energy. I have 4-ounce servings for breakfast or snack with fresh nuts on the side. It's usually 8 pieces of either almonds, walnuts, pecans, or a combination as a protein to maintain my blood sugar level.

I urge you to buy organic fresh fruits and veggies. Frozen fruits and vegetables are fine, but please make sure the package says organic. Foods that have been sprayed with chemicals are contaminated with highly toxic insecticides. You can find organic products in most markets, including box stores, at affordable prices.

Note: It is important to keep sugar levels low in your diet, and this is especially true with smoothies.

To your health!

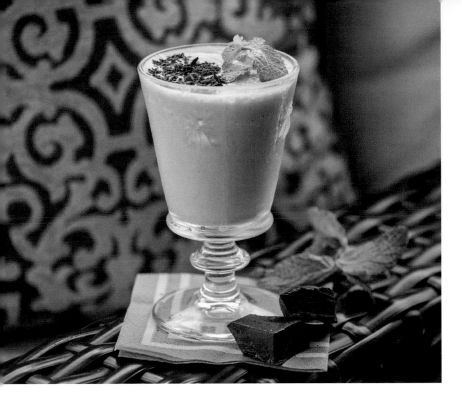

Matcha is loaded with antioxidants to a greater extent than fruits and vegetables. These antioxidants include a new variety called "catechins," which are found nowhere else. The catechin EGCg (or, epigallocatechin gallate) is believed to have properties that may help fight cancer.

SERVES 2

INGREDIENTS

1 cup unsweetened coconut milk

2 teaspoons matcha powder (this may seem like very little, but matcha tea is very potent)

½ cup low-fat Greek yogurt, plain

½ teaspoon Stevia

1 small organic banana

3 tablespoons rolled oats

½ cup baby spinach

10 ice cubes

3 mint leaves, torn into small pieces

1 teaspoon finely grated dark chocolate

INSTRUCTIONS

1. Place the coconut milk, matcha, yogurt, Stevia, banana, oats, spinach, and ice cubes into a blender. Blend on high for two minutes until smooth and creamy.

2. Pour into chilled glasses and top with the mint and chocolate!

Morning Matcha

I have a matcha smoothie at least 3 times a week and drink a cup of matcha tea every day. I do have a compromised immune system, and I know I'm providing its best defense by including matcha in my diet.

Matcha, or powdered tea, is made from leaves of green tea, making it a powerful source of antioxidants. It boosts your metabolism and burns calories. It detoxifies effectively and naturally while helping calm the mind and relax the body. Matcha is rich in fiber, chlorophyll, vitamin C, selenium, chromium, zinc, and magnesium. It also helps lower cholesterol and blood sugar.

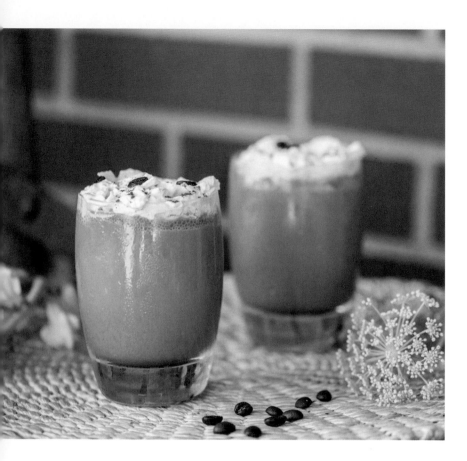

Polar Iced Coffee

MAKES 2¾ CUPS

INGREDIENTS

½ cup espresso or 1 cup strong brewed coffee, room temperature

12 organic coffee beans, whole

2 tablespoons unsweetened organic cocoa powder

1 small organic banana

16 ice cubes

⅓ cup hazelnut milk

1 tablespoon hemp seeds

2 tablespoons toasted hazelnuts, plus 1 tablespoon finely chopped toasted hazelnuts for garnish

½ teaspoon Stevia

2 heaping tablespoons dairy-free coconut whipped cream (found in the refrigerated section of your grocery store)

Pinch of ground cinnamon

INSTRUCTIONS

1. Pour the coffee, coffee beans, cocoa powder, banana, ice cubes, hazelnut milk, hemp seeds, 2 tablespoons hazelnuts, and Stevia in a blender on high speed for 1 minute.

2. Pour into a glass and top with the whipped coconut cream, reserved chopped hazelnuts, and the cinnamon.

Green Monster Power Booster

I find myself dragging around 4 o'clock every afternoon. If I don't eat or drink something to bring my energy level up to hold me until dinner, I will inevitably start picking—a piece of cheese here, tortilla chips there, pretzels, toast—you get the picture. I am committed to staying strong and healthy, so my choice is to make this delicious and good for you power-boosting smoothie. It gives me just the kick I need to continue on with my day, feeling strong and in control. This smoothie is great for breakfast too. I see green and automatically know it is good for me!

SERVES 2

INGREDIENTS

1 half avocado, peeled and pitted

1 small frozen banana

½ cup fresh spinach

2 cups chopped fresh or frozen pineapple

1 cup almond milk

¼ teaspoon Stevia

2 teaspoons chia seeds

2 teaspoons hemp seeds

16 ice cubes

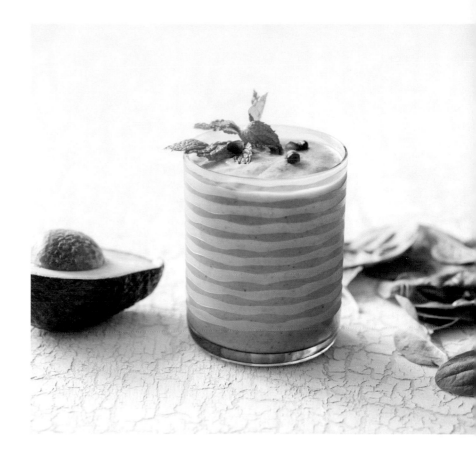

INSTRUCTIONS

Place the avocado, banana, spinach, pineapple, almond milk, Stevia, chia seeds, hemp seeds, and ice cubes in a blender. Process for 1 minute until the mixture is smooth.

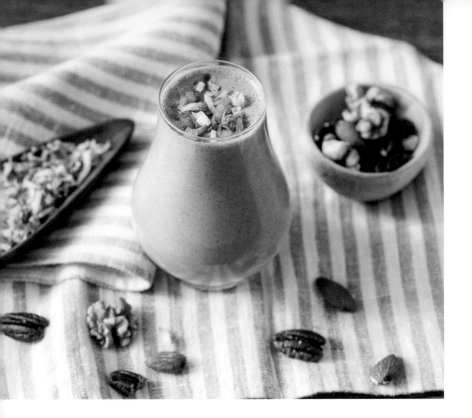

This Is Nuts!

I particularly love walnuts and eat them every day. I put them in my smoothies, salads, and snacks. Nuts are packed with protein and most contain heart-healthy unsaturated fats. The good fats in nuts lower bad cholesterol levels, and are loaded with antioxidants that can help you lose weight and reduce inflammation. Research shows walnuts may support brain health, and also enhance cognitive and motor function in those who are aging. Walnuts are rich in vitamin E, folate, melatonin, and omega-3 fats.

SERVES 2

INGREDIENTS

1 small banana

8 almonds, 8 walnuts, and 8 pecans

1 tablespoon organic chunky peanut butter

1 tablespoon cacao powder

10 ice cubes

1 cup unsweetened almond-coconut milk

1 tablespoon hemp seeds

1 tablespoon pure maple syrup

¼ teaspoon ground cinnamon

½ cup shredded coconut, toasted (see Toasted Coconut, p. 221)

INSTRUCTIONS

1. Place the banana, nuts, peanut butter, cacao powder, ice cubes, almond coconut milk, hemp seeds, and maple syrup in a blender; process for a one minute until smooth.

2. Pour into glasses and top each with ⅛ teaspoon cinnamon and a helping of toasted coconut.

Smooth Move

SERVES 2

INGREDIENTS

2 cups coconut water
½ cup oatmeal
1 small papaya, peeled, seeded, and cut into chunks
1 cup chopped fresh or frozen pineapple
2 teaspoons coconut extract
1 tablespoon flax seeds
1 tablespoon bran flakes
1 teaspoon chia seeds
2 teaspoons hemp seeds
¼ teaspoon Stevia
16 ice cubes
1 small banana, sliced
Pinch of freshly ground nutmeg and ground cinnamon
4 fresh mint leaves

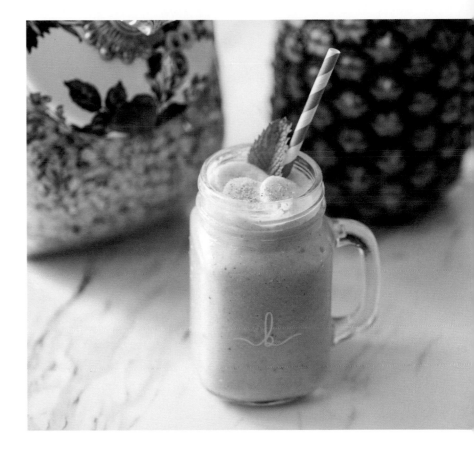

INSTRUCTIONS

1. Pour the coconut water over the oatmeal and let it sit 15 minutes at room temperature.

2. In a blender combine the oatmeal mixture, papaya, pineapple, coconut extract, flax seeds, bran flakes, chia seeds, hemp seeds, Stevia, and ice cubes. Blend for 1 minute or until it's smooth and creamy.

3. Pour into glasses, and evenly divide the sliced banana, cinnamon, nutmeg, and garnish with two leaves of mint for each serving.

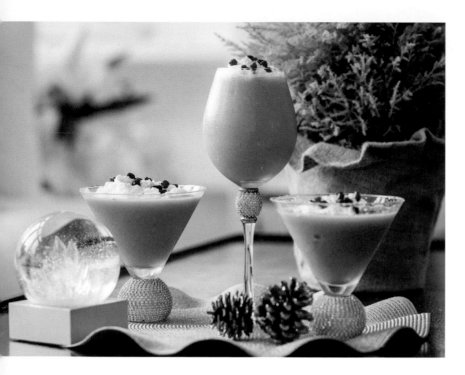

Holiday Cheer

I serve this smoothie during the holiday season to my family and guests. Just because it may be cold outside doesn't mean you can't enjoy this heart-healthy drink that includes the star of the season—pumpkin! I usually have this pumpkin smoothie for dessert instead of sweets. Pumpkin is filled with potassium, fiber, and vitamin C, all of which support heart health.

Here's a little secret for the grown-ups: if you want to add rum and go sit by the fire, I highly suggest that! One ounce per serving should do the trick. Happy Holidays!

SERVES 4

INGREDIENTS

2 small bananas

1 cup pure pumpkin, canned (*not* the pie filling)

1 cup fresh orange juice

1 teaspoon ground cinnamon, plus more for garnish

½ teaspoon ground nutmeg, plus more for garnish

¼ teaspoon Stevia

12 ice cubes

4 tablespoons dairy-free coconut whipped cream

1 tablespoon pomegranate seeds

1 tablespoon orange zest

INSTRUCTIONS

1. Place the banana, pumpkin, orange juice, cinnamon, nutmeg, Stevia, and ice cubes into a blender and process 1 minute until it's smooth.

2. Pour into chilled glasses and garnish with the whipped cream, pomegranate seeds, orange zest, cinnamon, and nutmeg! Serve immediately.

Dreaming of the Tropics

SERVES 4

INGREDIENTS

1 small organic banana

2 cups chopped fresh or frozen pineapple

½ cup fresh orange juice

1 cup (5 ounces) mango, chopped into pieces

1 cup canned or boxed coconut cream

¼ teaspoon Stevia

2 teaspoons coconut extract

1 tablespoon fresh lime juice

3 fresh mint leaves

16 ice cubes

4 strawberries

4 fresh mint sprigs

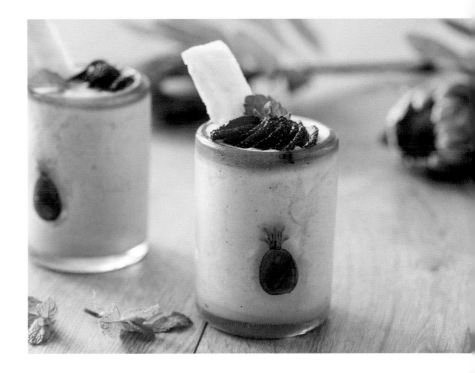

INSTRUCTIONS

1. Place the banana, pineapple, orange juice, mango, coconut cream, Stevia, coconut extract, lime juice, mint leaves, and ice cubes into a blender. Blend on high for 2 minutes or until it's smooth and creamy.

2. Pour into chilled glasses and garnish each serving with the strawberries and mint.

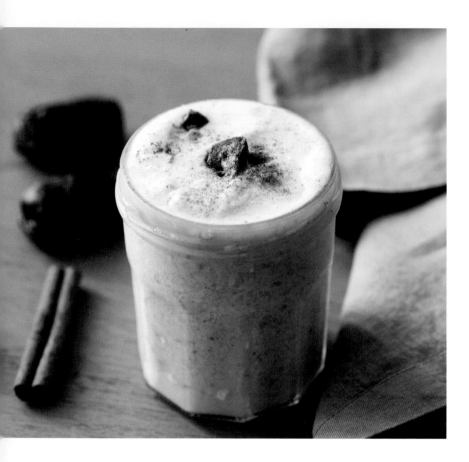

Date Me!

SERVES 4

INGREDIENTS

2 cups unsweetened almond-coconut milk
8 pitted Medjool dates
½ cup low-fat Greek yogurt, plain
1 tablespoon pure maple syrup
½ teaspoon cinnamon plus more for garnish
20 ice cubes
½ cup chopped pecans, plus 4 whole pecans for garnish

INSTRUCTIONS

1. Combine the almond-coconut milk, 6 dates, yogurt, maple syrup, cinnamon, ice cubes, and chopped pecans in a blender. Blend on high for 1 minute until it's smooth!

2. Chop the extra 2 dates. Garnish each serving with of pinch of cinnamon, a pecan, and divide the chopped dates among the drinks.

Berry Smooth Energy Boost

Adding chia, hemp, or flax seeds to any smoothie is one of the best things you can do to insure you are getting the health benefits of omega-3s in your diet. I also sprinkle chia and hemp seeds in salads, soups, and sandwiches.

Chia seeds are one of the richest plant-based sources of omega-3s (the others being flaxseed, hemp seeds, and walnuts). They provide a large quantity of phosphorous, calcium, and fiber as well. Omega-3s may help to lower LDL cholesterol, triglyceride, and blood pressure. They also may reduce atherosclerotic plaque build-up in your arteries.

MAKES 3½ CUPS

INGREDIENTS

6 strawberries, hulled and rinsed

1 cup raspberries, plus ¼ cup for garnish

1 small organic banana

½ cup low-fat Greek yogurt, plain

½ teaspoon Stevia

¾ cup cashew, coconut, or almond milk

1 teaspoon chia seeds

1 teaspoon hemp seeds

16 ice cubes

6 fresh mint leaves

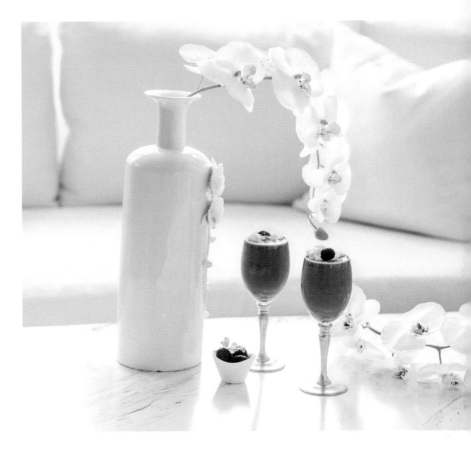

INSTRUCTIONS

1. Combine the strawberries, 1 cup raspberries, banana, yogurt, Stevia, nut milk, chia seeds, hemp seeds, and ice cubes in a blender. Process on high for 1 minute until smooth.

2. Pour into glasses and top with the remaining ¼ cup raspberries. Garnish with the mint.

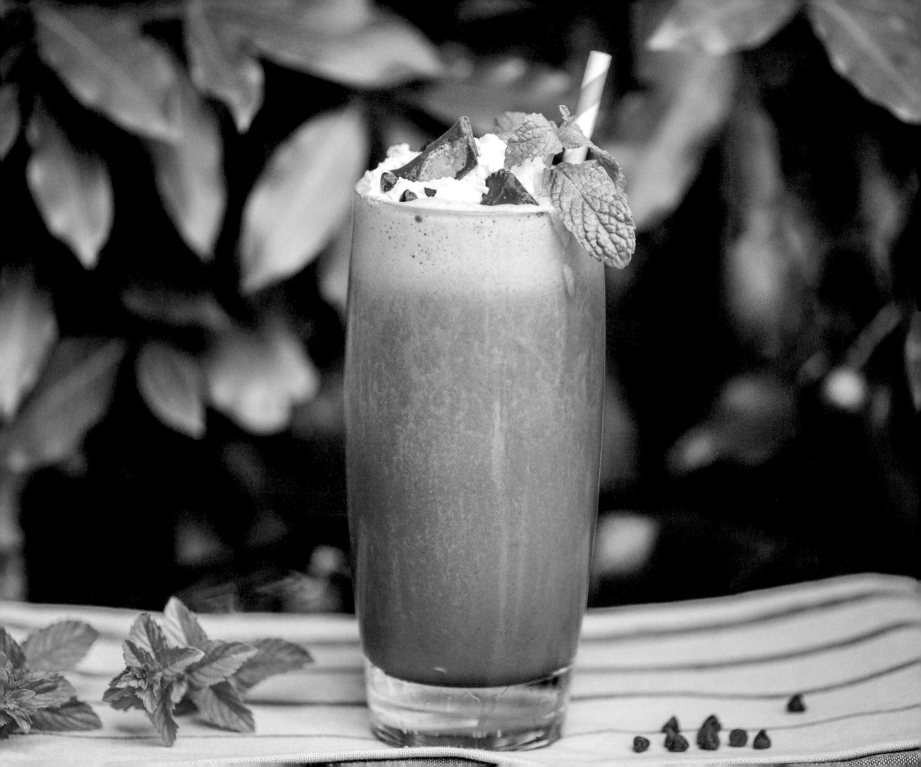

Peanut Butter and Chocolate!

My one guilty pleasure all my life has been eating peanut butter cups. My problem was (and still is) that I wouldn't eat just one package. No, I ate at least three packages that contained two peanut butter cups in each serving at one sitting. So, if you do the math, that's six cups. I loved it while I was eating them, but I paid the price afterwards. There was an immediate high from the sugar, the usual dull throbbing headache that accompanied it, an aching tummy, followed by a "crash," and then I turned into Ms. Crabby Patty.

I'm happy to say that I don't do that anymore. I just don't like the way I feel afterwards. So I have a choice: Do I want unnecessary fat and added sugar in my body and the way it makes me feel, or do I want to enjoy them in a way where I get the same satisfaction with the added bonus of ingredients that are good for me? I found a way to combine my two favorite ingredients, chocolate and peanut butter, into one smoothie.

Let's stay realistic here—bananas and natural peanut butter **do** *contain natural sugar, so I limit the portions to 4-ounce servings. I still benefit from the natural ingredients and get the satisfaction of a truly delicious drink that makes me happy!*

SERVES 4

INGREDIENTS

2 small bananas, cut one into ¼-inch slices for garnish

¼ cup organic crunchy peanut butter

2 cups hazelnut, coconut, or cashew milk

3 tablespoons unsweetened cacao powder

2 teaspoons vanilla extract

½ teaspoon Stevia

16 ice cubes

1 cup dairy-free whipped cream

4 miniature peanut butter cups, cut in half

2 teaspoons organic mini chocolate chips

4 fresh mint leaves

INSTRUCTIONS

1. Place 1 banana into a blender and add the peanut butter, your choice of nut milk, cacao powder, vanilla extract, Stevia and ice cubes. Blend for 1 minute until smooth and creamy.

2. Pour into chilled glasses and garnish each serving with a dollop of dairy-free whipped cream, 2 slices of banana, 1 peanut butter cup half, and sprinkle on ½ teaspoon mini chocolate chips. Garnish with the mint on top.

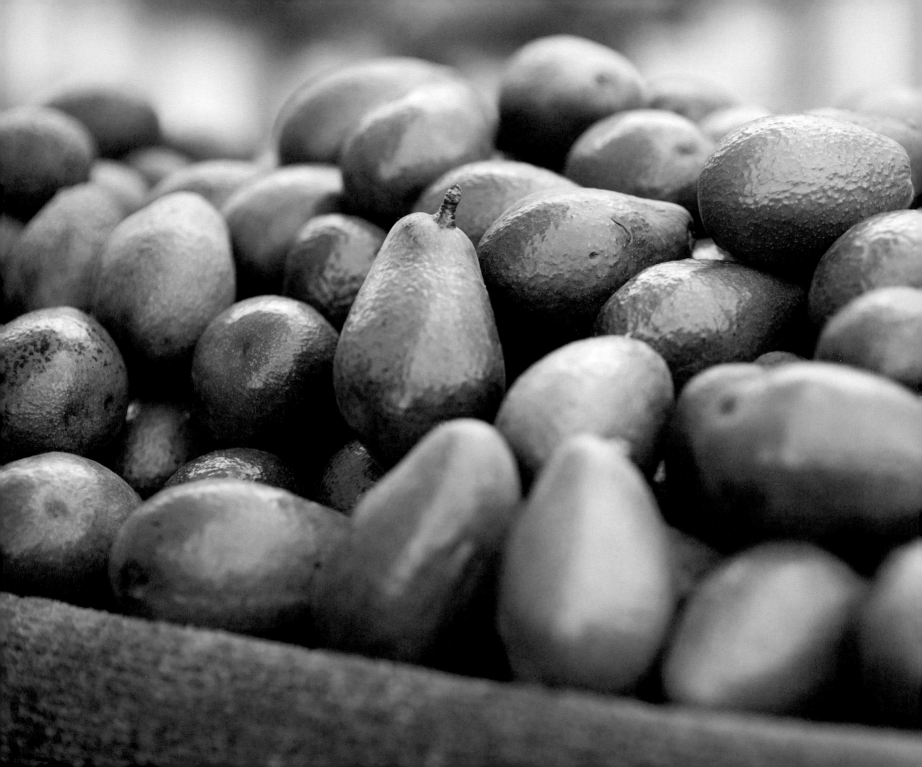

Salads & Veggies: A Garden of Earthly Delights

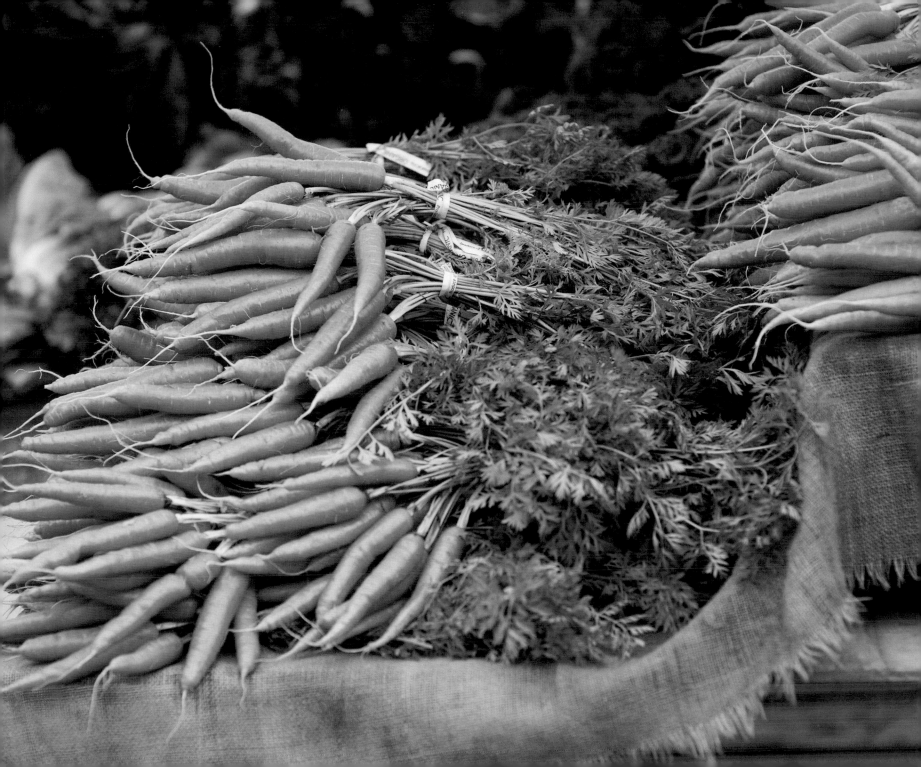

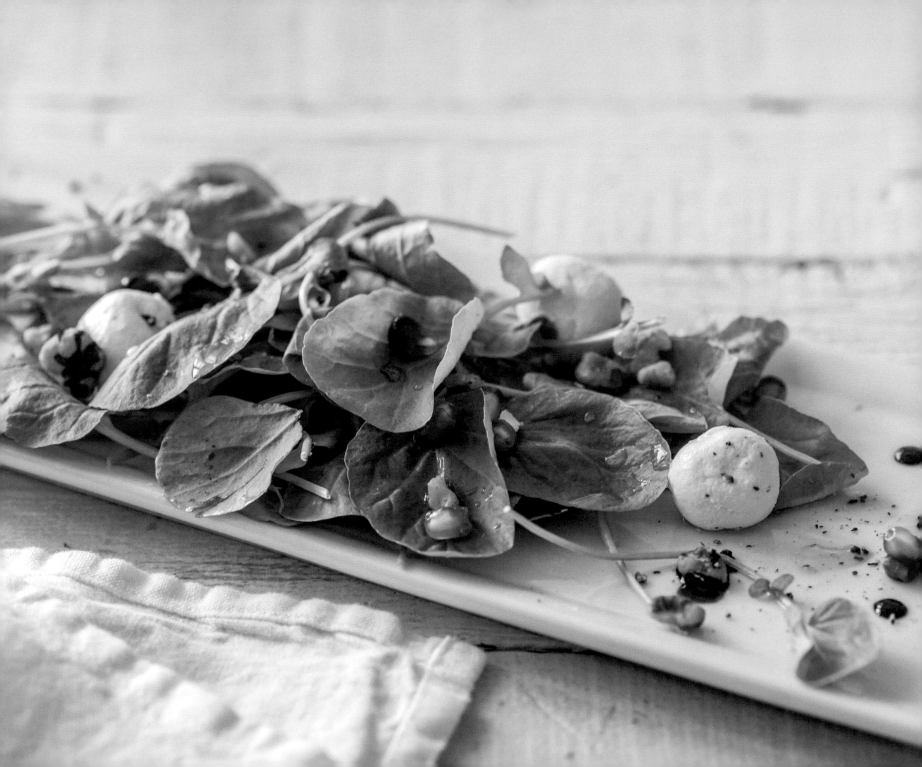

Watercress Salad

THE #1 SALAD GREENS
YOU SHOULD EAT OFTEN!

You should know that not all greens are created equal. I eat a lot of salads with different kinds of lettuce and greens in them, and I was surprised when I learned that the top-rated salad green is watercress! It contains the highest percentage of your daily recommended intake for vitamins K, A, B$_6$, B$_{12}$, D, E, C, calcium, iron, and magnesium. It scored 106 percent on the CDC's density score of 0 to 100. This green cruciferous veggie is on the list of cancer-fighting foods, helps build strong bones, and is important for eye health.

*The CDC determines the nutritional density of greens by looking how they fulfill daily requirements for nutrients for your body including potassium, fiber, protein, calcium, iron, thiamin, riboflavin, niacin, folate, and zinc. Interestingly, my research found that **eight** salad greens are ranked in the top.*

I was so happy to read this since I'm a huge lover of watercress with its peppery bite. I add it to many of my salads and as a topping for sandwiches, grilled dishes, and soups to wake up their flavors!

SERVES 2

INGREDIENTS

2 bunches watercress

Creamy Shallot Vinaigrette (see recipe, p. 208)

2 tablespoons crumbled Greek or French feta cheese,
    or 10 goat cheese balls rolled into ½-inch pieces

2 tablespoons pomegranate seeds

2 tablespoons finely chopped walnuts

INSTRUCTIONS

1. To prepare the watercress, Hold the watercress by its stems upside down. Using a sharp knife, start at the bottom of the stem and gently pull the knife down to cut the leaves off. Do this all around; some of the stems will remain.

2. Gently rinse the watercress well in cold water and spin dry to remove the water off its tender leaves. Place the cleaned and dried watercress in a salad bowl.

3. Drizzle 3 tablespoons Shallot Vinaigrette over salad and mix gently. Arrange the watercress between two plates and divide the feta or goat cheese, pomegranates, and walnuts between the two plates.

Chopped Garden Salad

Making this raw vegetable chopped salad is something I do often. I get a mega dose of nutrients and vitamins that carry me through the whole day, and I love that it is raw, which preserves every nutrient.

Eating more fruits and vegetables as part of an overall healthy diet is likely to have reduced risk of some chronic diseases, such as type 2 diabetes and certain cancers, such as stomach and colon. It may also help reduce risk of coronary heart disease, kidney stones, and help to decrease bone loss. Vegetables provide nutrients that are vital for health and maintenance of your body.

SERVES 6 TO 8

INGREDIENTS

3 cups baby arugula, coarsely chopped

3 cups baby spinach, coarsely chopped

2 small zucchinis, diced

1 small- to medium-sized red, orange, and green bell pepper, each seeded and diced

2 carrots, peeled and diced

4 celery ribs, diced

1 cucumber, seeded and diced

20 organic cherry or small Roma tomatoes, halved

1 cup Monterey Jack cheese, cut into small cubes, or 1 cup crumbled Greek feta

1 (15-ounce) can organic garbanzo beans, drained and rinsed well

1 teaspoon kosher salt

5 tablespoons dressing (see Chapter 10 for a variety of vinaigrette options)

¼ cup fresh mint leaves, coarsely chopped

¼ cup fresh basil leaves, coarsely chopped

INSTRUCTIONS

1. In a large wooden salad bowl, begin by arranging the arugula in a pile on one side of the bowl in a triangle shape. Then place the remaining Ingredients the same way all around the bowl packed tightly next to one another. It will end up looking like a colorful pinwheel! Mix the salad at the table so everyone can see how beautiful it looks!

2. Sprinkle the salt over the salad and drizzle it with the dressing. Sprinkle on the fresh mint and basil, mix, and serve!

Cook's Note: If you find there are other vegetables you like better, such as roasted corn, artichoke hearts, kale, and so forth, use those. And for any veggie you don't like, just substitute your choice. The same with beans, if garbanzos don't do it for you, try cooked navy, black, or kidney beans. You can also add 1½ cups roasted or grilled chicken breast, grilled or boiled shrimp, or tofu cut into ¼-inch cubes.

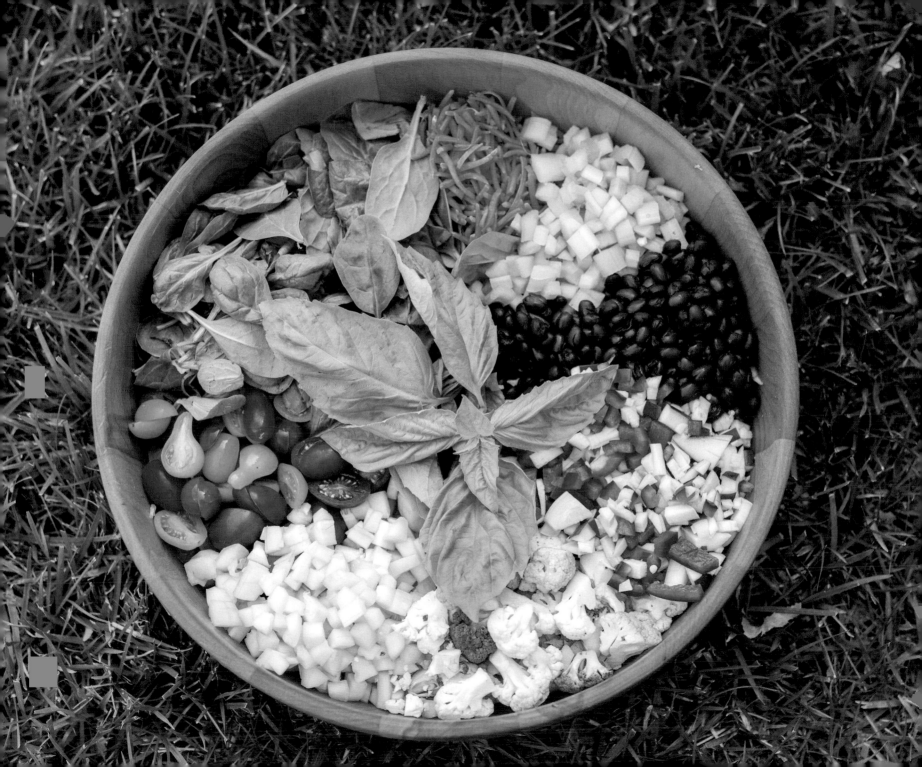

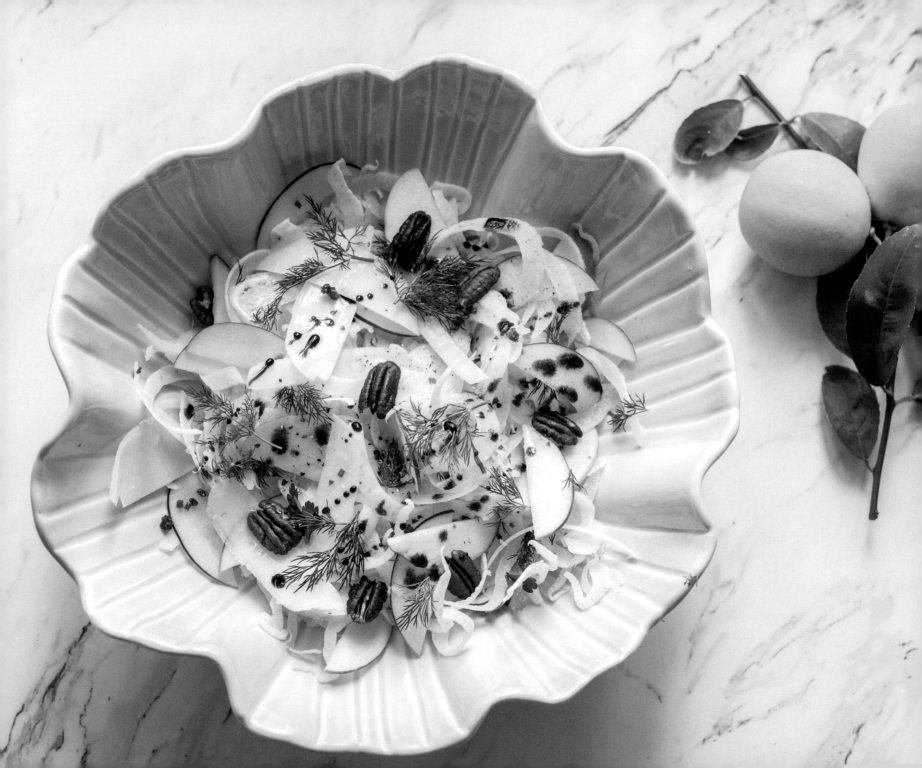

Shaved Fennel, Apple, Parmesan Cheese, and Fresh Herbs Salad

There are many health benefits of fennel including relief from anemia, indigestion, flatulence, constipation, colic, diarrhea, respiratory disorder, and menstrual cramps. Fennel fiber supports heart health with high contents of potassium, folate, and phytonutrients. Coupled with its lack of cholesterol, fennel helps decrease the risk of heart disease. When you make this salad don't forget to add the long fronds above the fennel bulb because those contain a number of important vitamins, such as vitamins D and B_6.

Sweet fennel has a hint of anise flavor, so adding fresh lemon juice and a good green olive oil brings out its clean, almost fruity flavor. Using slightly salty Parmesan cheese and the clean, bright tartness of the green apples is a perfect mix of flavors refreshing to the palate.

SERVES 4

INGREDIENTS

2 large fennel bulbs, sliced thinly on a mandoline to yield about 4 cups

1 green apple, cored and sliced on a mandoline to 1/8-inch thickness

1/2 teaspoon kosher salt and cracked black pepper

10 mint leaves, coarsely chopped

Lemon Vinaigrette (see recipe, p. 213)

1 1/2 cups shaved Parmesan cheese

4 sprigs fresh dill, leaves only

8 to 10 fennel fronds

20 whole pecans

4 lemon wedges

Balsamic Glaze, store-bought or homemade (see recipe, p. 212)

INSTRUCTIONS

1. Scatter the fennel in a serving bowl, and add the apple, salt, pepper, and mint. Add 1/3 cup Lemon Vinaigrette and toss together. Adjust the seasoning by adding more salt to taste. Serve with lemon wedge on the side.

2. Scatter the Parmesan cheese, dill, fennel fronds, and pecans on top. Drizzle Balsamic Glaze over the top.

Tip: Sprinkle 2 tablespoons lemon juice over the apple slices to keep them from turning brown

Watermelon Salad

Sweet summer watermelon is one of my favorite fruits ever! Who doesn't look forward to an ice-cold slice of watermelon on a hot, sticky, humid July or August day!

I had always thought that this sweet indulgence offered nothing in terms of nutritional value, until I found out this refreshing fruit, which is mostly water, about 92 percent, is loaded with nutrients. Each juicy bite has significant levels of vitamins A, B_6, and C, lots of lycopene, antioxidants, and amino acids. There's even a modest amount of potassium.

One of my favorite ways to eat watermelon these days is an icy cold watermelon salad with small chunks of coarse sea salt, thinly sliced onion, feta cheese, fresh mint, a good green olive oil, and a drizzle of Balsamic Glaze. The cold, sweet, juicy watermelon absorbs all the distinct flavors of those ingredients and brings a most satisfying palate-pleasing experience.

SERVES 6

INGREDIENTS

1 (5–6 pound) seedless watermelon, cut into six 2-inch slices

6 tablespoons extra-virgin olive oil

18 (1-inch) thick square slices Greek or French feta cheese

4 thin slices red onion, separated into rings

6 sprigs of mint

½ cup microgreens

Balsamic Glaze, store-bought or homemade (see recipe, p. 212)

TO ASSEMBLE

1. Place a slice of the melon on a very clean chopping board. Using a knife, slice the rind off the top, bottom, and sides so you have a perfect 4½-inch square of watermelon.

2. Slice off any rind you see remaining on the edges. Finish cutting the rest of the watermelon into squares.

3. Stack all the pieces together and wrap tightly in plastic wrap. Refrigerate for 2 hours or more.

4. For each serving, place one slice of watermelon on a serving plate and make three horizontal cuts, 1½-inches apart then 4 vertical slices 1½-inches apart. You should have 9 squares per serving.

5. Place 3 pieces of feta and 4 to 5 individual rings of onion on each plate of melon. Drizzle 1 tablespoon olive oil all over. Break off pieces of the mint sprigs and garnish the top of the melon.

6. Drizzle Balsamic Glaze and scatter microgreens over the top. Serve immediately.

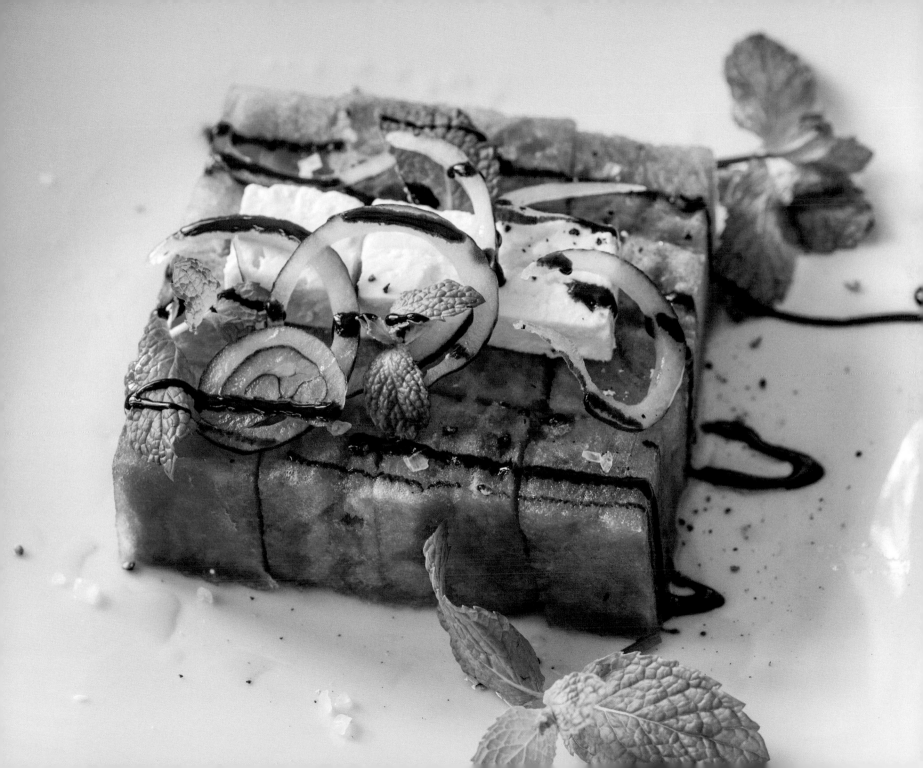

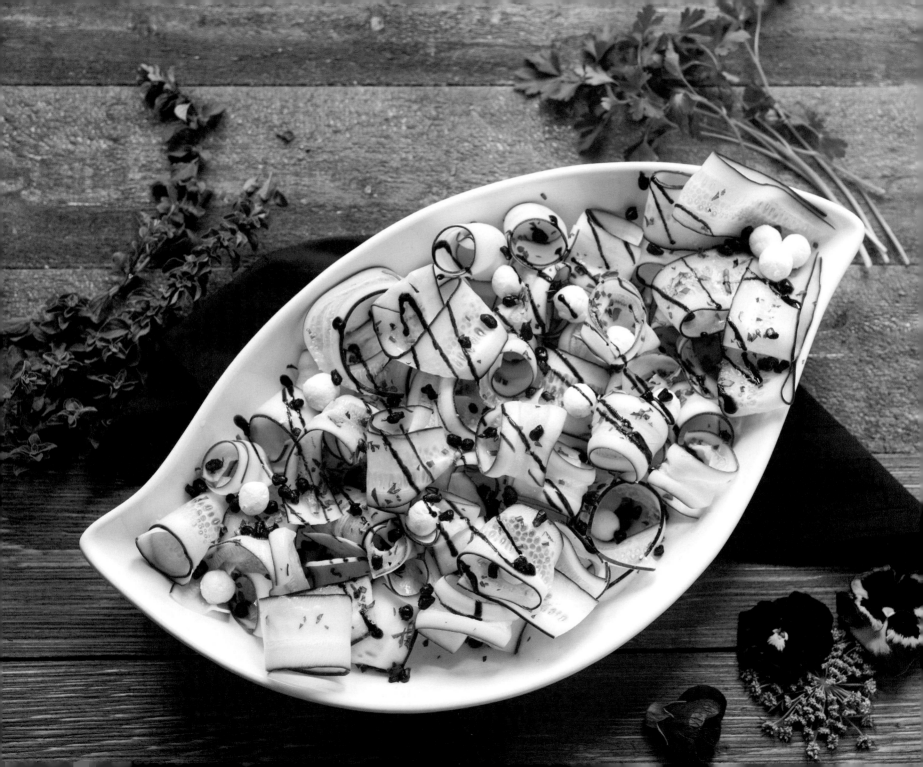

Cucumber and Zucchini Carpaccio with Fresh Herbs

SERVES 4 TO 6

INGREDIENTS

2 large zucchini, cut into ¼-inch lengthwise ribbons on a mandoline

2 cucumbers, cut into ¼-inch lengthwise ribbons on a mandoline

½ cup crumbled Greek or French feta cheese

2 tablespoons fresh mint, finely chopped

2 tablespoons chopped fresh dill

¼ cup finely chopped roasted walnuts

Cracked black pepper

⅓ cup fresh raspberries or pomegranate seeds

Raspberry Vinaigrette (see recipe, p. 209)

Balsamic Glaze, store-bought or homemade (see recipe, p. 212)

INSTRUCTIONS

1. Fill a large bowl with 1 quart water and add 3 cups ice.

2. Loosely roll the zucchini and cucumber slices around your index finger, secure each with a toothpick, and place them in the bowl of ice water. It's okay if any unravel a bit. Cool in the refrigerator for 1 hour.

3. To prepare the salad

4. Drain the zucchini and cucumber in a colander and lay them on paper towels to air dry for 20 minutes.

5. Remove each toothpick and arrange the zucchini and cucumbers like ribbons on a large platter. Scatter the feta, mint, dill, and walnuts on top. Season with the pepper.

6. Drizzle 5 tablespoons Raspberry Vinaigrette over the vegetables, scatter raspberries or pomegranate seeds on top, and drizzle the Balsamic Glaze over all.

Note: If you are not going to serve the salad right away, do not add the Raspberry Vinaigrette or the Balsamic Glaze. Instead, cover with plastic wrap and refrigerate until you are ready to serve.

Avocado Citrus Salad

This salad is a sensory overload work of art. Extremely appealing to the eye, the taste is refreshing and clean, and the aroma is fresh and citrusy. The combination of citrus with the creaminess of avocado, and the peppery taste of arugula work together beautifully.

In California, citrus fruits are available all year long. I always have bowls filled with these fruits in my kitchen, and use them in many dishes. Citrus contain several different antioxidants that may help prevent diseases such as heart disease and cancer, and even skin damage from the sun. Grapefruit juice may help lower blood pressure. In addition to fiber and vitamin C, citrus fruits supply calcium, potassium, folate, and vitamin A.

SERVES 4

INGREDIENTS

1 bunch (2 cups) prepared watercress

4 cups baby arugula, rinsed well and spun dry

1 large white grapefruit, peeled and sectioned

1 large navel orange, peeled and sectioned

2 medium ripe avocados, peeled, pitted, and cut into ½-inch slices

3 tablespoons fresh lemon juice

28 red grapes, sliced

4 thin slices red onion, separated into rings

1 cup Italian (flat leaf) parsley, coarsely chopped

20 fresh mint leaves, coarsely chopped

⅓ cup pomegranate seeds

Honey Poppy Seed Dressing

20 whole Toasted Walnuts (see recipe, p. 221)

⅛ teaspoon each of kosher salt and cracked black pepper

INSTRUCTIONS

1. In one hand, tightly hold the watercress upside down at the bottom of their stems. With your other hand, angle the blade of a knife and gently pull down to remove the leaves from the stems. Do this until most the leaves have been separated from their stems. Discard the stems. Wash the watercress well and spin dry.

2. Place the arugula in a salad bowl and add the prepared watercress. Toss well. Divide the greens between four plates.

3. For each serving split equally grapefruit and oranges, alternating the fruit as you place them over top of salad greens.

4. Lift half of one of the sliced avocados and place it on the side of the salad plate. Gently press down on the avocado slices to fan them out.

5. Over each plate, scatter 14 grape halves, 5 walnuts, several red onion rings, ¼ cup parsley, the mint, and several pomegranate seeds.

6. Drizzle 2 to 3 tablespoons of the Honey Poppy Seed Dressing over the top of each plate. Sprinkle with the salt and pepper.

Tip: Squeeze lemon juice over the avocado slices to keep them from turning brown.

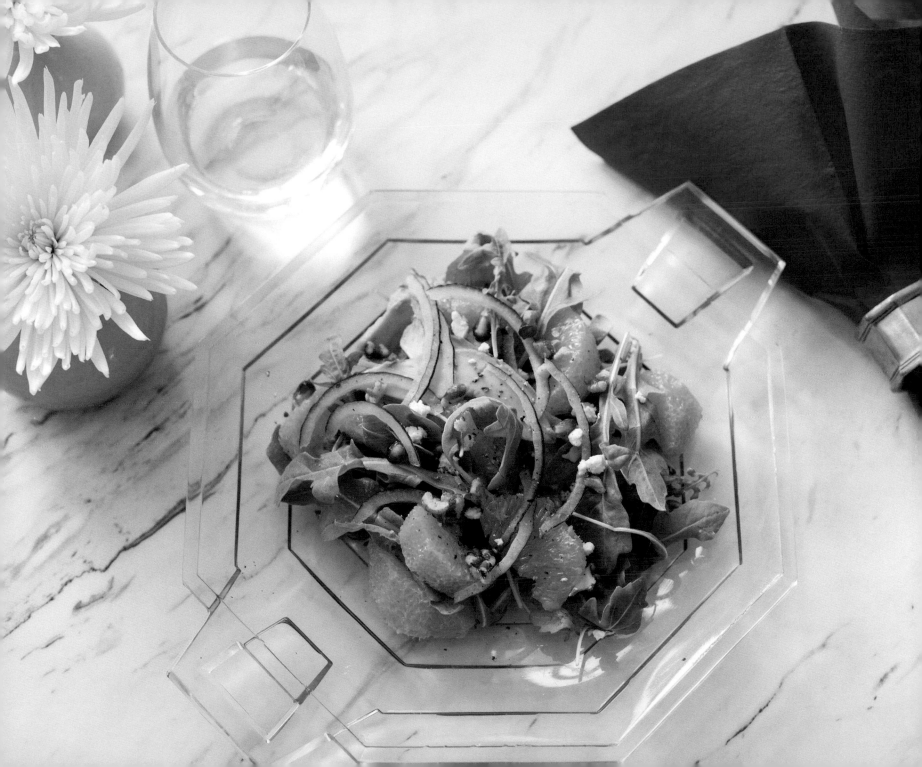

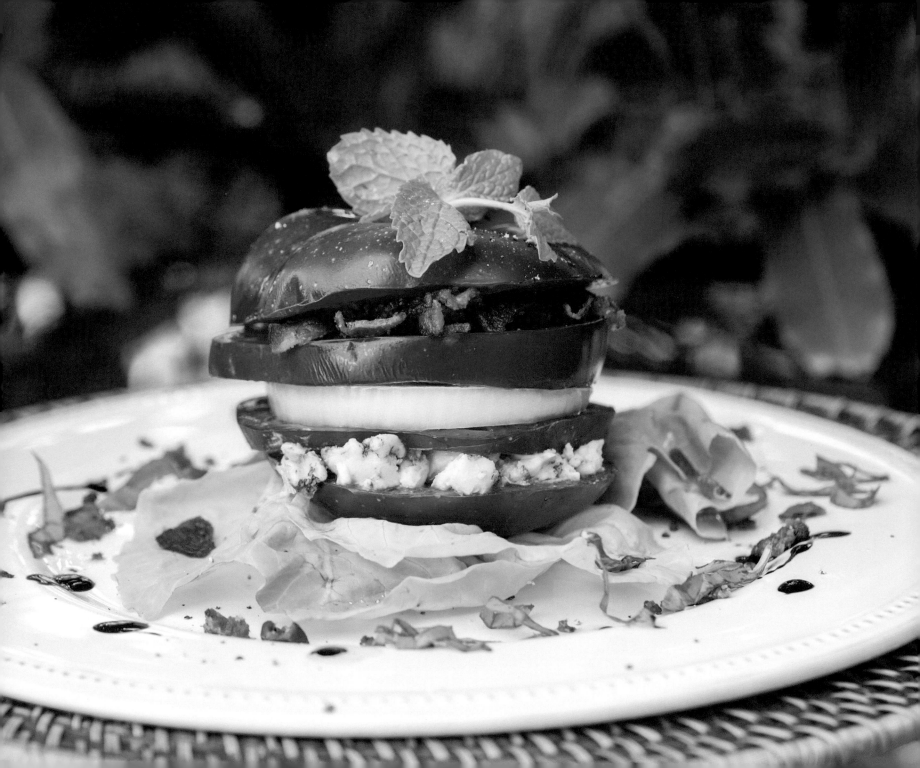

New Twist on the Wedge Salad with Creamy Blue Cheese Dressing

My husband is obsessed with wedge salads dripping with blue cheese dressing! I decided to invent a recipe that he will love, be heart-smart, and won't clog his arteries! This salad is typically made with iceberg lettuce, which is made up of 95 percent water, contains only small amounts of fiber and minerals, and is devoid of any nutritional value.

So, instead of the iceberg lettuce I use a large organic tomato, full of heart-healthy lycopene; a snappy white onion, important for cell growth and division; the best quality blue cheese for the dressing; and butter lettuce.

There is scientific evidence that blue cheese may help lower the risk of cardiovascular disease, as well as lower cholesterol levels and help prevent blood clots. It has anti-inflammatory properties that will reduce artery inflammation, joint inflammation, and arthritis pain.

SERVES 4

INGREDIENTS

1 head Bibb lettuce, leaves separated, rinsed in cool water, and spun dry

4 medium uniformly sized organic tomatoes

Blue Cheese Dressing (see recipe, p. 210)

1 small white onion, sliced into ¼-inch-thick rounds

10 basil leaves

4 strips uncured nitrate-free bacon, cooked until crispy, drained, and crumbled into small chunks

Small chunks pink Himalayan salt

Balsamic Glaze (see recipe, p. 212)

4 tablespoons extra-virgin olive oil

INSTRUCTIONS

1. Arrange 3 to 4 Bibb lettuce leaves on each of the 4 salad plates.

2. Stack the basil leaves on top of each other, roll tightly into a cylinder, slice thin, and set aside.

3. Using a serrated knife, slice a small round piece off of the bottom of each tomato so it will stay stable on the plate. Slice the rest of each tomato in 4 even slices.

4. For each serving, place a slice of tomato in the middle of the Bibb lettuce, sprinkle with a pinch of salt, and add just enough Blue Cheese Dressing to cover the first layer.

5. Place the second tomato slice over the dressing and add an onion slice.

6. Place the third slice of tomato on top and add 3 to 4 basil thins over, several pieces of crumbled bacon. Add last slice of tomato.

7. Garnish with more basil strips, leftover bacon bits, and scatter 3 to 4 chunks of the Himalayan pink salt all around.

8. Drizzle top and sides of plate with Balsamic Glaze. Drizzle 1 tablespoon each of olive oil over the top of each tomato and plate.

9. Serve with extra Blue Cheese Dressing on the side.

Quinoa Bowl

I use quinoa just like any other grain such as rice or barley. I boil it in either in chicken or vegetable broth. I make beautiful healthful salads, with quinoa and use it as a bed for chicken, stews, fish, or beef dishes. Quinoa can also be used in casseroles and enjoyed for breakfast as a porridge with fresh fruit and nuts! It is gluten-free, high in protein, and popular among vegetarians and vegans, because all nine essential amino acids are contained within these tiny grains. It is high in fiber, magnesium, vitamins B and E, iron, potassium, calcium, phosphorus, and various other beneficial antioxidants.

Be sure to rinse quinoa really well because the grains have a coating that can make it taste bitter. Even if the package says pre-rinsed, I still rinse it.

4 TO 6 SERVINGS

INGREDIENTS

1 cup quinoa
1 mango, peeled and diced
1 red bell pepper, seeded and diced
1 small cucumber, peeled, seeded, and diced
1 cup shelled edamame
3 scallions, white and light green part, finely chopped
⅓ cup sliced almonds
⅓ cup raisins or dried cranberries
1 Gala apple, skin on, cored, and cut into bite-sized pieces
¼ cup coarsely chopped Italian (flat leaf) parsley
1 teaspoon each kosher salt and cracked black pepper
⅓ cup Balsamic Vinaigrette (see recipe, p. 211)
1 tablespoon lime zest
8 fresh basil leaves, rolled tightly and sliced into thin ribbons

INSTRUCTIONS

1. In a large saucepan cook the quinoa according to package directions, rinse in cool water, drain in a mesh strainer and shake out as much water as you can.

2. Place the drained quinoa in a large serving bowl. Add the mango, bell pepper, cucumber, edamame, scallions, almonds, raisins or cranberries, apple, parsley, salt, and pepper.

3. Add the Balsamic Vinaigrette, salt, and pepper and toss gently. Top with the lime zest and basil ribbons!

Cook's Tip: One cup of dry quinoa will yield 3 cups when cooked. It usually takes 2 cups of liquid to 1 cup quinoa and about 20 minutes to cook. Don't forget to add ¼ teaspoon kosher salt to each cup of dried quinoa during cooking.

Tip: Squeeze 1 tablespoon fresh lemon juice over the apple pieces to prevent them from turning brown.

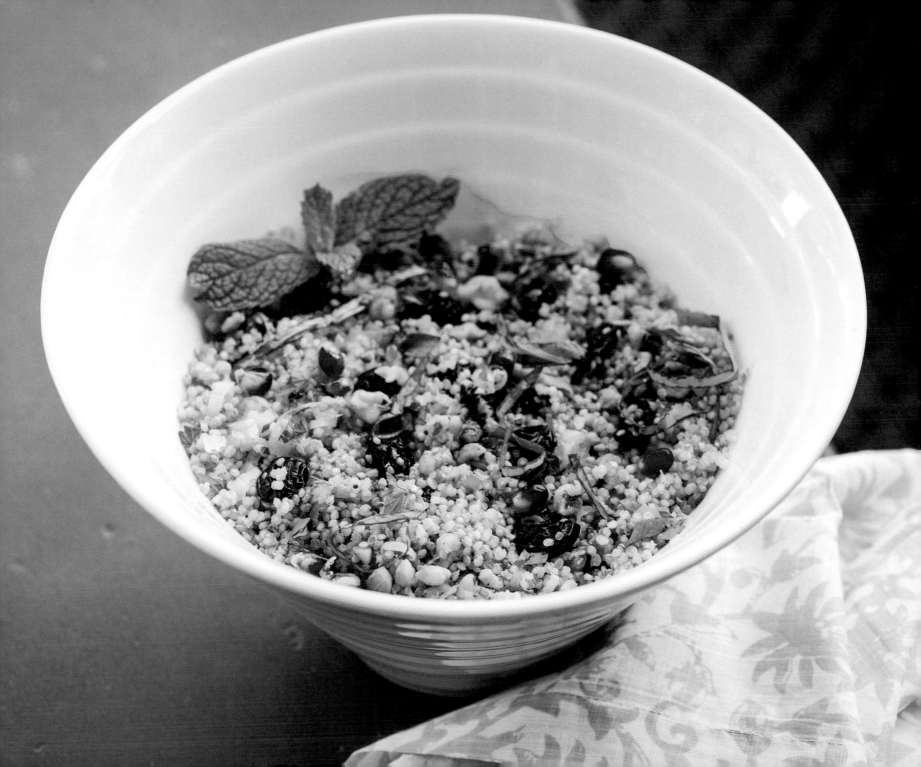

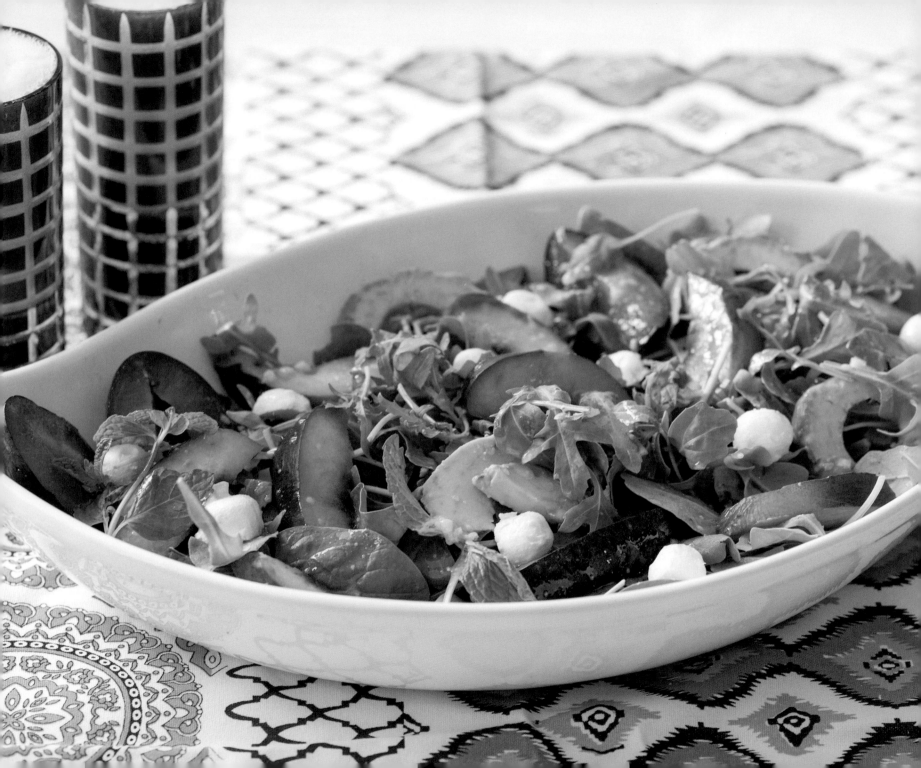

Stone Fruit Salad

Eating stone fruits is part of a healthy diet and you can enjoy them on their own or in combination with other ingredients—like this beautiful salad! Peaches and other stone fruits are high in potassium, which is essential for muscle function. Apricots support heart health and eye function. Plums contain antioxidants that fight off free radical damage, protect the skin, and promote good health. Cherries contain antioxidants, fiber, and potassium, and studies suggests that the antioxidants can help improve circulation and are anti-inflammatory.

SERVES 6

INGREDIENTS

4 cups organic baby arugula

3 cups organic baby spinach

¼ cup fresh mint leaves, torn

½ cup fresh basil, coarsely chopped

2 plums (not overly ripe), pitted and quartered

2 peaches, pitted and quartered

4 small apricots, pitted and quartered

1 cup fresh cherries, pitted and sliced in half

2 medium avocados, peeled, pitted; cut each half into thirds

Goat cheese rolled into 12 grape-sized balls

Citrus Vinaigrette (see recipe, p. 210)

Kosher salt and cracked black pepper

¼ cup coarsely chopped walnuts

INSTRUCTIONS

1. On a large serving platter scatter the arugula, spinach, mint, and basil all over the bottom.

2. Place the plums, peaches, apricots, and cherries on top of the greens. Arrange the avocado slices. Scatter the goat cheese balls.

3. Drizzle 5 to 6 tablespoons of the Citrus Vinaigrette over everything. Finish with a sprinkle of salt and pepper and walnuts. Keep extra dressing available on the side for anyone who would like more!

Tip: Squeeze 1 tablespoon fresh lemon juice over the avocado slices to prevent them from turning brown.

Caesar Salad with Creamy Dressing and Homemade Croutons

The first time I ordered a Caesar salad, it was my first experience in a "big girl" restaurant. As I watched the waiter made the salad tableside, I loved it until I saw him drop a raw egg yolk into the dressing! I sat with the salad in front of me and wouldn't touch it, even though the aroma made my mouth water. I couldn't get past the raw egg yolk—still can't. The raw yolk was to help make the dressing creamy. No thank you!

You can still get that smooth almost silky consistency without the raw yolk by combining the dressing ingredients in a blender until emulsified.

The second ingredient I struggled with were the anchovies. When anchovies are used in sauces and dressing they impart a salty, slightly fishy flavor, but when I tasted it I loved the way all of the ingredients worked together to create a dressing that was rich in flavor. Three anchovy fillets are enough to season about 1 cup of Caesar salad dressing. I've grown to love anchovies as does my whole family. I always lay extra strips of them over the salad. It's a good thing, too, because they contain omega-3 fatty acids, which help build strong bones. There are benefits to the heart as well, with essential B vitamins, and they are a rich source of iron.

SERVES 6

INGREDIENTS

6 romaine hearts (the center leaves of romaine lettuce)
1½ cups freshly grated Parmesan cheese
1 (2-ounce) can anchovy fillets in olive oil
Cracked black pepper
1 lemon cut into quarters
Ceasar Dressing (see recipe, p. 211)
Croutons (see recipe, p. 222)

INSTRUCTIONS

1. Rinse the romaine hearts in cool water and use a salad spinner to spin dry. If you don't have a salad spinner roll each romaine heart in paper towels and pat dry.

2. For each serving, stack the romaine lettuce leaves on a plate to make it look like a full head. (See photo.)

3. Drizzle 3 to 4 tablespoons of the Caesar Dressing over the romaine. Scatter 6 to 8 croutons over each salad, sprinkle 3 tablespoons of the Parmesan cheese, and top with 2 anchovy fillets. Add some of the cracked black pepper over and serve with a lemon wedge on the side.

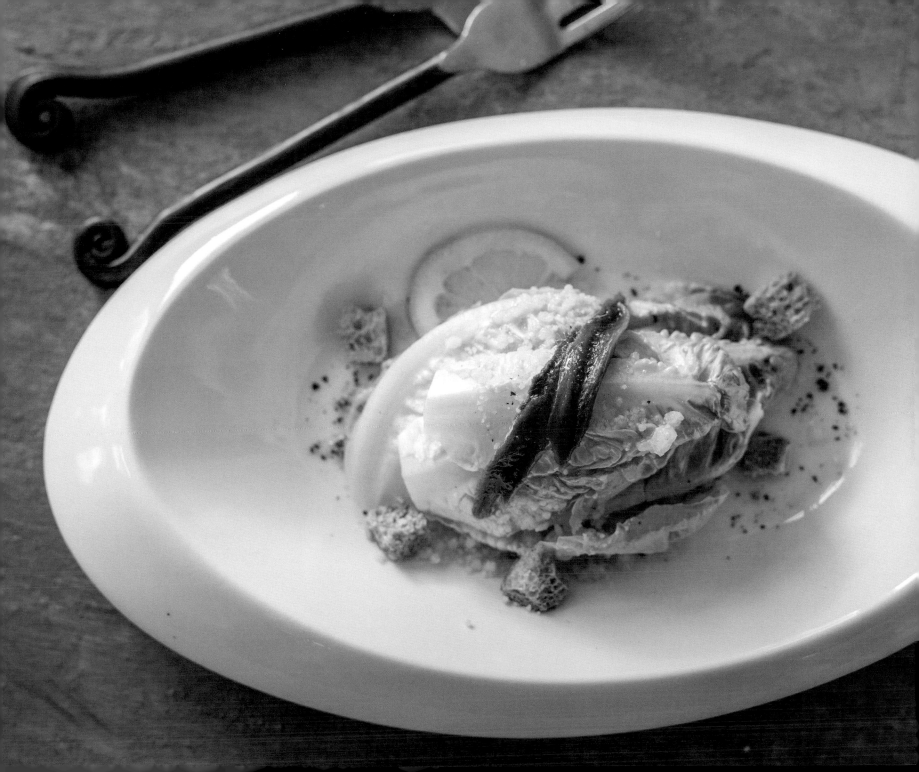

Body Healing Salad

Did you know that there are foods that actually look like parts of your body? We are going to do a little exploring, and I will show you exactly what I mean. We'll start at the top of your head and travel through your body to show you the benefits of those certain foods for particular parts of your body! It's amazing to see and to learn about it!

BRAIN

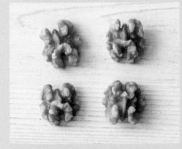

If you look at the folds and wrinkles of a walnut you can clearly see that its shape resembles that of the human brain. It even looks like it has a left and right hemisphere.

Walnuts have a very high content of omega-3 fatty acids, which support brain function. Many studies have been shown that adding walnuts to your daily diet improves memory and overall cognitive function.

Walnuts can significantly help lower cholesterol and research shows walnuts to be promising in the fight against cancer. Research also has found that just a few walnuts per day may help reduce blood pressure. With all of the stress that we face from day to day it's just one of the natural ways to help lower it.

EYES

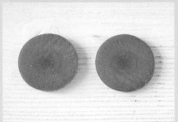

We all know that carrots contain vitamin A and you should include them in your diet to help promote healthy eyes. Slice a carrot in half crosswise and you can clearly see that the vegetable resembles the eye! Look at the photo—you can actually see the pupil and the iris! This is crazy! I love it!

Carrots are filled with vitamins and antioxidants like beta-carotene, which help decrease the chance of macular degeneration, which is the leading cause of vision loss in the elderly. The retina of the eye needs vitamin A to function. A study found that people who eat foods rich in beta-carotene had a 40 percent lower risk of macular degeneration.

HEART

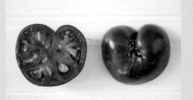

When you slice open a tomato you can actually notice multiple chambers that look like the structure of a heart!

Tomatoes contain lycopene which can help reduce the risk for heart disease in men and women. Just one serving of a red, ripe raw tomato is a great source of vitamins A, C, K, folate, and the important B$_6$ vitamin. It helps relieve stress, which is always good for the heart, brain, and body. Stress in the body directly affects the brain and causes damage and, little by little, you start to literally lose your mind.

STOMACH

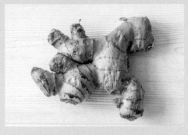

Ginger root looks like a stomach. It has been used for thousands of years as a digestive aid and cure for tummy troubles.

It helps treat nausea, fights fungal infections, protects against stomach ulcers, eases menstrual pains, and may inhibit cancer growth.

I steep a piece of ginger root in hot water every day, and I feel the warm, soothing effect it has on me immediately. Ginger contains a phytochemical that can help prevent nausea and vomiting. The word "phytochemical" refers to the compounds found in plants that are extremely beneficial protecting humans from disease.

PANCREAS

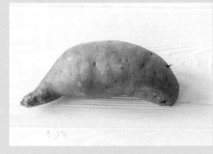

Sweet potatoes resemble the pancreas and promote healthy function of this organ. The sweet potato is high in beta-carotene, which as we discussed is a powerful antioxidant and helps protect tissues in the body from damage associated with the aging process.

They are anti-inflammatory and filled with antioxidants! Inflammation is the enemy of the body. So it is important to eat foods that keep toxins out of your system. It is considered a "super food" filled with high amounts of vitamins A, C, and B.

UTERUS

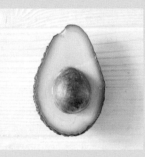

Avocados resemble a uterus (the womb), and they support reproductive health. Folic acid, folate, (there are those important and vital B's again) is the key for cell growth, which is important for pregnant women. Avocados have potassium and vitamins C and E.

I eat a small avocado every day by itself or on toast or in salads, and I also blend them in smoothies!

CELLS

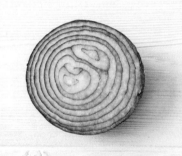

When you cut open an onion you can see they look like cells in the body. Here are just a few of the incredible health benefits of the onion!

Research shows onions clear waste materials from body cells. Onions have chromium, which assists in regulating blood sugar. They also contain vitamin C, which helps improve immunity and reduces inflammation. It lowers the bad cholesterol (LDL) and therefore helps you keep a healthy heart. Onions eat away at free radicals in the body. We want that!

BONES

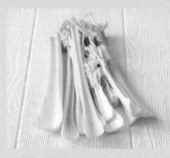

Celery stalks are shaped like bones and the mineral silicon, a main source of bone strength, is significantly involved in collagen production. Dietary silicon must be replenished as we age to maintain healthy bones. Silicon promotes he hair, helps smooth damaged skin, and improves brittle nails.

Women begin to lose bone mass after age 30, so it's never too early to begin your bone health program. Don't forget cardio exercise 30 minutes a day to get oxygen to the brain and light weightlifting to maintain strong bone health.

HEART AND TESTICLES

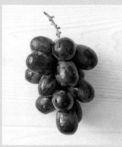

If you look at grapes hanging in a cluster it resembles the shape of the heart and also testicles.

Resveratrol found in the skin of red grapes reduces inflammation and is vital in the prevention of testicular and prostate cancer. Resveratrol also makes it more difficult for platelets to stick together and form clots, one of the many ways to help prevent heart attacks. Resveratrol helps lower LDL cholesterol (bad cholesterol). Red wine is rich in antioxidants & polyphenols including powerful resveratrol.

Grapes are helpful in enhancing the health of the brain and delaying the onset of diseases like Alzheimer's. The polyphenols in grapes have been found to reduce cognitive decline associated with the disease.

Body-Healing Salad

I have assembled all of the body-healing vegetables described in this section and created a delicious salad. It literally feeds specific parts of your body to enhance your overall health! Make the Asian Citrus Vinaigrette first, or pick a dressing from the Vinaigrettes and Salad Dressings chapter (see p. 207).

SERVES 2

INGREDIENTS

1 small sweet potato (dark orange inside), peeled and cut into ½-inch cubes

1 tablespoon extra-virgin olive oil

Kosher salt

1 grapefruit, peeled and sectioned

1 ripe avocado, peeled, pitted, and sliced into ½-inch-thick pieces

2 cups organic baby arugula

1 cup baby spinach, well washed

1 heirloom tomato, cored and sliced ¼-inch thick

2 carrots, peeled and sliced ¼-inch thick

2 celery ribs, sliced ¼-inch thick pieces

1 red onion, thinly sliced

12 whole toasted walnuts, recipe below

½ cup red grapes, sliced in half

2 fresh figs, each sliced open lengthwise, optional

Cracked black pepper

1 teaspoon sesame seeds

6 mint leaves
Asian Citrus Vinaigrette (see recipe, p. 210)
Toasted Walnuts (optional; see Tip)

INSTRUCTIONS FOR THE SWEET POTATO

1. Preheat the oven to 350F°.

2. Drizzle 1 tablespoon olive oil over the sweet potato and use your hands to coat the cubes. Add a pinch of kosher salt. Roast 20 to 30 minutes until the cubes are tender and have started to caramelize on the sides.

TO ASSEMBLE THE SALAD

1. Divide the arugula and spinach between 2 plates.

2. Add 3 to 4 tomato slices on each plate.

3. Alternate 3 slices each of grapefruit and avocado on top of the greens.

4. Scatter the sweet potato, carrots, celery, onion, walnuts, grapes, and a fig, if you're using figs.

5. Sprinkle kosher salt, cracked pepper, sesame seeds, and mint leaves over top of salad.

6. For each serving drizzle 2 to 3 tablespoons of the Asian Citrus Vinaigrette over the top of the salad.

Cook's Note: If figs are in season I highly recommend you add it to this salad. Figs lower triglycerides, are a natural remedy for ulcers, and are full of fiber, calcium, and potassium. *They are an antioxidant powerhouse!*

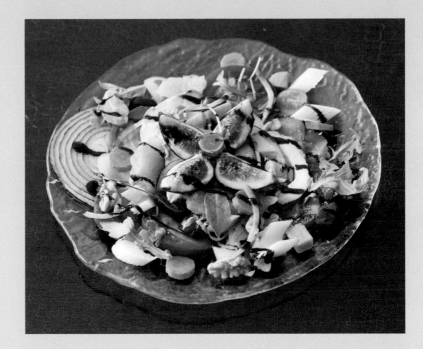

Tip: To toast the walnuts, place them in in a cold, dry frying pan and turn the heat to medium. Shake the pan back and forth every few moments until they start to release their oil and turn slightly brown, 3 to 4 minutes. Be careful not to burn them or they will taste bitter. (See Toasted Walnuts recipe, p. 221.)

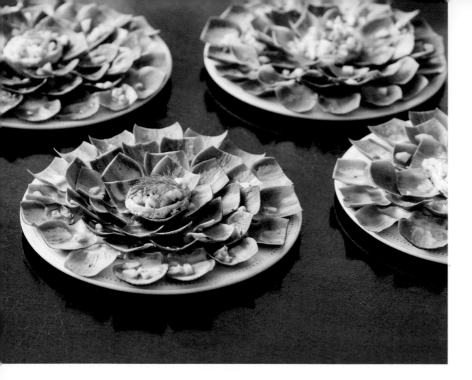

Bloomin' Artichokes

Artichokes are one of my favorite vegetables; I love them steamed and grilled! When in season from March through May, I have artichokes several times a week.

Did you know that artichokes are not actually a vegetable? They are a variety of thistle. That's what accounts for those annoying prickly things I always get stuck with when I am preparing them.

Here is the good part: artichokes are associated with the benefits of protection against various forms of cancer. They help boost your immune system, lower cholesterol, aid in digestion, and help with constipation and irritable bowel syndrome (IBS). Who knew?

Of course, I just can't put an artichoke in a bowl and pull the leaves off one by one and eat it. No, I have to create a visual experience as well! I love my artichoke flowers; they are not hard to do and the presentation is so beautiful. I know my family and guests appreciate the extra effort. Here's how to make them!

SERVES 6

INGREDIENTS

½ cup extra-virgin olive oil

2 tablespoons Dijon mustard

½ cup fresh lemon juice

1 tablespoon low-sodium soy sauce

2 tablespoons rice wine vinegar

¼ teaspoon kosher salt

2 scallions, white and light green parts, finely chopped

2 tablespoons finely chopped fresh Italian (flat leaf) parsley

3 tablespoons chopped fresh dill

2 tablespoons finely chopped fresh basil

1 tablespoon fresh mint, finely chopped

3 cucumbers, peeled, seeded, and diced small (set aside in a glass bowl)

6 large artichokes

INSTRUCTIONS

1. In a medium-sized glass bowl whisk the olive oil and Dijon mustard until it's homogenized. Whisk in the lemon juice, soy sauce, rice wine vinegar, salt, scallions, parsley, dill, basil, and mint. Pour over the cucumbers and mix together well. Season to taste by adding more salt if necessary.

2. Cover with plastic wrap and chill in the refrigerator for an hour or more.

TO ASSEMBLE

1. About an hour before you're ready to serve, fill a large bowl with ice water and squeeze the juice from 2 lemons into it. Set aside.

2. Using a serrated knife, cut off 2 inches from the top of the artichoke. Cut the stem so that the artichoke can stand on its own without tipping. Pull off the smaller leaves towards the base and on the stem, and discard. Use a scissors to cut off any excess thorns from the leaves. Place each artichoke in the lemon water after you are done prepping each one.

3. To cook, place the artichokes in a large pot and fill it with cold water to cover.

4. Bring the water to a boil on high heat. Reduce the heat to medium for a gentle boil. Cook 45 minutes and test for doneness by pulling off a couple of leaves and scraping them between your teeth to make sure they are soft. Cooking time depends on how large the artichoke is.

5. Another way to test for doneness is to take a small paring knife and insert it down the middle of the artichoke; if it slides in smoothly, they're ready.

6. Using tongs, lift the artichokes from the water and turn them upside down to drain. When they are cool enough to handle pull off all the leaves and place them in a bowl. You will be left with the "heart."

7. Now that the heart is exposed, use a sharp paring knife and on an angle, gently cut around the whole heart and gently lift out the middle, then discard. The heart is ready for the filling.

8. For each serving, place the heart in the middle of the plate and surround the heart with the artichoke leaves from the bowl. It will end up looking like a big, beautiful flower.

9. Fill the center of the heart with the Cucumber Vinaigrette plus scatter more of the vinaigrette all around the artichoke leaves.

Tip: You can prepare the artichokes and vinaigrette the day before and keep in the refrigerator until ready to assemble and serve.

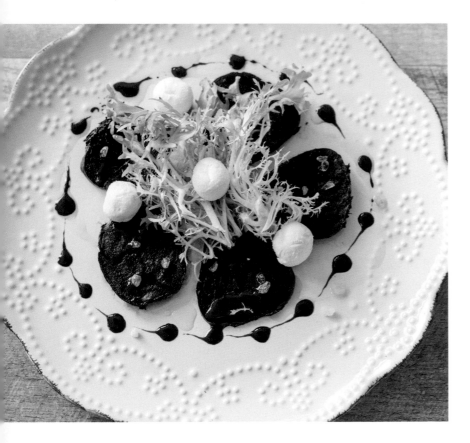

Caramelized Roasted Beet Salad with Goat Cheese

*I would **never** eat beets as a kid; I thought they tasted like dirt. It wasn't until I saw a recipe with roasted beets that I gave it another go. Roasting them brings out a sweet, earthy flavor after they caramelize. Pairing beets with a creamy goat cheese and finishing with Balsamic Glaze creates texture and a taste that is pleasing to my palate. Now Roasted Beets are always on my Sunday brunch menu! It's one of my favorite ways to prepare beets!*

Studies show that increasing consumption of plant foods decreases the risk of obesity, diabetes, heart disease, and increases energy. The health benefits of adding beets to your diet are significant. Beet root is a rich source of folate and manganese, along with vitamins B_6 and C, magnesium, potassium, zinc, copper, and selenium, which is important for cognitive thinking. Consuming beet juice can improve oxygen to the brain and slow signs of the progression of dementia in older adults. Beets can help boost longevity, and strength, improves digestion and improves sexual health.

SERVES 4

INGREDIENTS

3 tablespoons extra-virgin olive oil, divided

4 medium to large uniformly sized red or yellow beets, tops and ends cut off and scrubbed clean

4 cups frisée lettuce, washed and spun dry

¼ teaspoon kosher salt

20 grape-sized goat cheese balls

Champagne Vinaigrette (see recipe, p. 212)

½ cup chopped Toasted Walnuts (see recipe, p. 221)

Balsamic Glaze, homemade or store-bought (see recipe, p. 212)

INSTRUCTIONS

1. Preheat the oven to 425F°.

2. Pour 1 tablespoon olive oil in the palms of your hands and rub each beet all over to coat. Repeat as needed, using all the olive oil if necessary.

3. Place the beets on a baking pan and bake 1 hour and 15 minutes, or until tender. To check for doneness, insert a sharp paring knife through the middle of the thickest part of the beet. If the knife goes through all the way smoothly, the beets are done. Remove from the oven and cool completely.

4. Peel the beets under cool running water and cut them into ¼-inch slices.

5. In a small salad bowl add the frisée lettuce, salt, and 4 tablespoons of Champagne Vinaigrette dressing; toss together.

6. For each serving, arrange 5 beet slices in a circle on a salad plate. Place the frisée lettuce in the middle of the of the beets.

7. Arrange 5 goat cheese balls around the salad, and top with pieces of toasted walnuts.

8. Drizzle Balsamic Glaze over the beets. Add 1 to 2 teaspoons extra dressing, if you'd like.

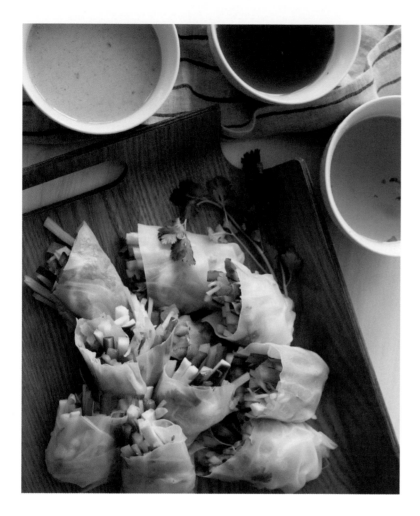

Vegetable Spring Rolls with 3 Dipping Sauces

One of my favorite ways to eat lots of raw, fresh, crunchy, colorful, flavorful vegetables is to roll them in rice paper. I end up eating 4 to 5 spring rolls at a sitting, they're that good! You are eating a virtual rainbow of colors! These little packages of mouthwatering goodness are packed with our daily requirements of vitamins and minerals, essential nutrients, antioxidants, and they have anti-inflammatory properties. I serve these spring rolls for lunch or dinner, as appetizers, as a snack, for a buffet, and during Sunday brunch!

I've added shrimp to this recipe, but you can also use tofu or grilled chicken. All of these proteins are optional. Also included are three dipping sauces, and while I don't know which one I like best, I just go to town enjoying the extra flavor power boost! I double the recipe for the sauces because I've actually seen people eating them with a spoon! Plus, I want my own serving on the side.

SERVES 6 TO 8

INGREDIENTS FOR THE SPRING ROLLS

12 medium raw shrimp, peeled, deveined, and tails removed (see Cook's Note)

1 bunch Thai or regular basil

12 cilantro sprigs

1 red bell pepper, seeded, sliced into thin strips

1 medium carrot, peeled, cut in half, sliced into thin strips

4 celery ribs cut in half, sliced into thin strips

1 cucumber, peeled, seeded, cut in half, sliced into thin strips

1 zucchini, ends trimmed off, sliced into thin strips

8 sheets rice paper (available in most markets), soaked

INSTRUCTIONS

1. Prepare a bowl of ice water to hold the shrimp after it has been boiled.

2. Bring 2 quarts of water to a boil and boil the shrimp for 2½ minutes. Drain the shrimp and place them in the ice water to stop them from cooking further for about 10 minutes. Cool. Slice each shrimp in half from top to bottom.

3. On a baking sheet, line up the shrimp pieces, basil, cilantro, bell pepper, carrot, celery, cucumber, and zucchini so they are side by side.

4. Fill a large flat-bottomed bowl or pie plate with warm water and add one sheet of the rice paper. Gently use your hands to immerse the whole paper. Lift it gently and place the wet rice paper on a clean cutting board.

5. On the lower third of rice paper lay 3 pieces of shrimp down crosswise, keeping the rice paper clear by 1 inch on each side. On top of shrimp add 3 basil leaves, 1 cilantro sprig, 4 to 5 strips bell pepper, and a few strips each of carrot, celery, cucumber, and zucchini.

6. Roll the rice paper tightly over the filling once. Tuck each side to seal, continue to roll tightly until you have formed a cylinder. Slice each spring roll on the diagonal and serve with dipping sauce.

Tip: If you wish to serve the spring rolls at a later time, tightly wrap them in plastic wrap and refrigerate until ready to serve.

Cook's Note: To peel and devein raw shrimp, start underneath where the legs are attached. Hold the shrimp firmly by its tail and pull off the shell, leaving the tail intact. Make a shallow slit down the middle of the back; you will see the black intestine. Under running water remove the intestine by lifting out the black vein. Use your hands to pull it out. Turn the shrimp over and do the same with the underbelly, removing the white vein.

Recipe continues, 3 Dipping Sauces ▶

3 Dipping Sauces

PEANUT VARIATION

INGREDIENTS

½ cup smooth peanut butter

2 tablespoons freshly grated ginger

4 tablespoons water

1 tablespoon seasoned rice vinegar

3 tablespoons fresh lemon juice

2 teaspoons sweet chili sauce

2 teaspoons light soy sauce or gluten free

1 teaspoon monk fruit

¼ teaspoon red pepper flakes

¼ teaspoon kosher salt

INSTRUCTIONS

1. Combine all ingredients in a blender and puree until smooth. If sauce is too thick, add more water, 1 tablespoon at a time, to reach creamy consistency.

2. Serve at room temperature!

SPICY VARIATION

INGREDIENTS

1 cup water

¼ cup seasoned rice vinegar

¼ cup fish sauce

1 tablespoon finely grated carrot

1 teaspoon monk fruit sweetener

1 garlic clove, peeled and crushed

½ teaspoon crushed red pepper

INSTRUCTIONS

In a small bowl stir the water, rice vinegar, fish sauce, carrot, monk fruit, garlic, and crushed red pepper.

GINGER VARIATION

INGREDIENTS

¾ cup water

2 teaspoons cornstarch

1 teaspoon monk fruit sweetener

2 tablespoons low-sodium soy sauce

½ cup seasoned rice vinegar

1 tablespoon fresh ginger, grated

½ teaspoon crushed red pepper

1 garlic clove, crushed

INSTRUCTIONS

1. In a small pot over medium-high heat, whisk the water and cornstarch until they're combined and no lumps are visible. Add the monk fruit, soy sauce, rice vinegar, ginger, crushed red pepper, and garlic. Bring to a boil and continue to cook until it thickens.

2. Remove from the heat and cool to room temperature.

Tip: Sauces can be refrigerated in tightly sealed glass containers for up to 3 days.

Hasselback Sweet Potatoes

Aren't these beautiful! I love sweet potatoes, and this is one of my favorite ways to prepare them. The skin is crispy and the insides are smooth, creamy, and sweet. I always have sweet potatoes in my pantry. They make delicious soups, salads, and desserts (such as my Chocolate Mousse, see p. 190), and of course, these delicious Hasselback Sweet Potatoes on their own!

One sweet potato contains 400 percent of your daily vitamin A requirement and has high amounts of fiber and potassium. The high fiber content helps prevent constipation and promotes regularity for a healthy digestive tract. It reduces chronic inflammation, which we need for gut health, and is considered low on the glycemic index scale. A sweet potato with its skin contains only 100 calories.

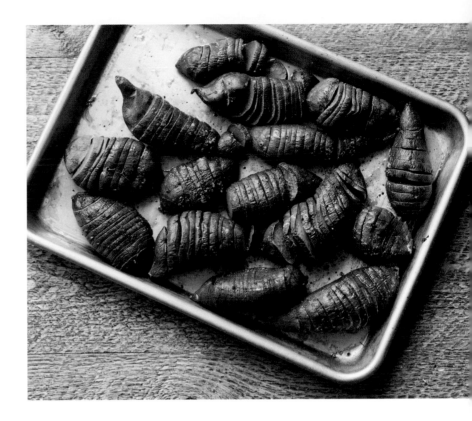

SERVES 6

INGREDIENTS

6 (1 pound total) sweet potatoes
⅓ cup extra-virgin olive oil
Kosher salt and cracked black pepper

INSTRUCTIONS

1. Preheat the oven to 425F°.

2. Slice a thin portion off one side of each potato and place the potato, cut flat side down, on a cutting board. Cradle a pair of chop sticks or wooden spoons on each side of a potato and Scotch tape them well to the board.

3. Use a sharp knife to make ⅛-inch-thick slices, cutting down to the chop stick or wooden spoon *but not through* the sweet potato. Place each prepared sweet potato on a baking sheet.

4. Using a pastry brush, lightly brush each potato with the olive oil. Season well with salt and pepper.

5. Bake 30 to 40 minutes until the sweet potatoes are golden brown and crispy.

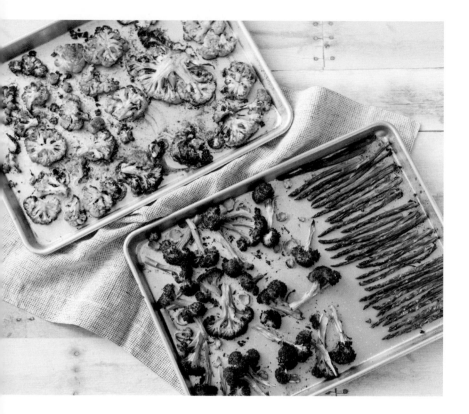

Roasted Cauliflower, Asparagus, and Broccoli

I like to roast all of these vegetables at once and serve them at the same time. Roasting is one of the healthiest methods to prepare vegetables since it uses dry heat to soften and then crisp the vegetables. The natural sugars from the vegetables are released when they are roasted and they end up tasting sweet and have a lovely crunch! I actually have to hide them, because if I leave them out before I'm ready to serve, they disappear.

ROASTED CAULIFLOWER

SERVES 4 TO 6

INGREDIENTS

1 large cauliflower, washed, dried, trimmed, and sliced into ¾-inch "steaks"

¼ cup extra-virgin olive oil

1 teaspoon onion powder

1 teaspoon garlic powder

2 teaspoons ground cumin

1 teaspoon turmeric

1 teaspoon kosher salt and cracked black pepper

⅛ teaspoon cayenne pepper

1 tablespoon lemon zest

1 tablespoon minced Italian parsley

Balsamic Glaze, (see recipe, p. 212)

INSTRUCTIONS

1. Preheat the oven to 450F°.

2. Lay the cauliflower steaks on a large baking sheet.

3. In a small glass bowl combine the olive oil, onion powder, garlic powder, cumin, turmeric, salt, pepper, and cayenne pepper. Mix well. Use a pastry brush to coat both sides of the cauliflower with the olive oil mixture.

4. Bake 20 to 30 minutes or until the cauliflower has caramelized and is crusty on top and bottom.

5. Garnish with lemon zest, parsley, and Balsamic Glaze.

ROASTED ASPARAGUS

INGREDIENTS

2 bunches asparagus, trimmed and woody ends snapped off

3 tablespoons extra-virgin olive oil

½ teaspoon kosher salt

2 lemons, cut into wedges

Balsamic Glaze, store-bought or homemade (see recipe, p. 212)

INSTRUCTIONS

1. Preheat the oven to 450F°.

2. Place the asparagus on a baking sheet in a single layer. Pour the olive oil over the asparagus, using your hands to coat each stalk. Add salt. Roast 20 to 30 minutes until caramelized and crispy.

3. Squeeze the lemon wedges over the asparagus just before serving.

4. Drizzle Balsamic Glaze over the top of all vegetables.

ROASTED BROCCOLI

INGREDIENTS

2 cloves garlic, peeled and smashed

¼ cup extra-virgin olive oil

⅛ teaspoon crushed red pepper

2 large heads broccoli, cleaned and cut into florets; stems cut into ¾-inch rounds

½ teaspoon kosher salt and cracked black pepper

INSTRUCTIONS

1. Preheat the oven to 450F°.

2. Place the garlic, olive oil, and crushed red pepper in a small bowl; let it sit for 30 minutes.

3. Toss the broccoli florets and stem rounds in the olive oil mixture. Place them on a baking sheet, and sprinkle with the salt and pepper.

4. Roast 20 to 30 minutes until they start to turn brown and get crispy around the edges.

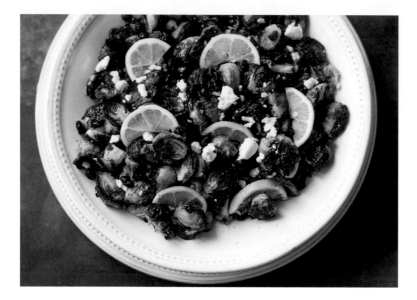

Roasted Caramelized Brussels Sprouts with Balsamic Glaze

I roast Brussels sprouts until they are deeply caramelized and crispy, it brings out their sweet, nutty flavor.

One serving of Brussels sprouts meets the daily requirements for vitamins C and K. They are low in fat and a great source of calcium, which is essential to bone strength and growth.

Freezing fresh Brussels sprouts does not harm them. They still maintain their flavor and nutrients, so you can enjoy them whenever you want throughout the year. I prefer freezing them myself, rather than buying them packaged frozen.

SERVES 8 TO 10

INGREDIENTS

2 pounds Brussels sprouts, trimmed and halved lengthwise; reserve any loose leaves

4 tablespoons extra-virgin olive oil, plus more for drizzling

1½ teaspoons each of kosher salt and cracked black pepper

½ cup pomegranate seeds

½ cup crumbled Greek or French feta cheese

Balsamic Glaze, homemade or store-bought (see recipe, p. 212)

1 lemon, sliced into thin rounds, each round cut in half

INSTRUCTIONS

1. Preheat the oven to 400F°.

2. In a bowl, combine the Brussels sprouts halves along with the loose leaves, olive oil, salt, and pepper; toss until coated. Place the Brussels sprouts on a baking sheet.

3. Bake 20 to 30 minutes or until the bottoms of the sprouts have caramelized and the tops have crisped.

4. Use a metal spatula to remove the Brussels sprouts and put them in a serving bowl. Cool 15 minutes; add the pomegranate seeds and feta.

5. Drizzle with the Balsamic Glaze and olive oil, and top with the lemon slices!

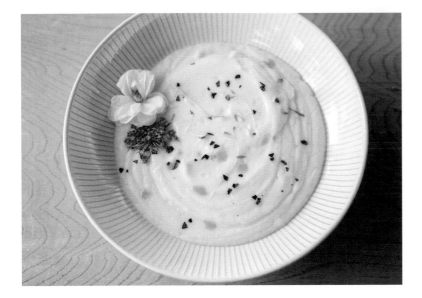

Cauliflower Purée with Hemp Oil

SERVES 4 TO 6

INGREDIENTS

1 large head cauliflower, cut up
2 garlic cloves, peeled and smashed
1 tablespoon extra-virgin olive oil
1 tablespoon kosher salt
2 tablespoons caper juice
2 teaspoons hemp oil (see Cook's Note)
1 teaspoon black salt, available online, or large-flake sea salt
1 small handful pea shoots or microgreens
Edible flowers

INSTRUCTIONS

1. In a stockpot cover the cauliflower with water by 2 inches. Add the garlic, olive oil, and salt. Bring to a boil for 15 minutes or until the cauliflower is soft and tender.

2. Drain the cauliflower and garlic (reserving 1 cup of cauliflower water). Place the cauliflower into a blender and add the garlic, caper juice, and ½ cup of the cauliflower water. Blend for 30 seconds.

3. Pour the cauliflower mixture into a saucepan and heat over medium-high heat. If you see that it is too thick, add more of the cooking water 2 tablespoons at a time.

4. Transfer the cauliflower to a vegetable bowl to serve and drizzle the hemp oil over the top. Sprinkle with the black salt, and garnish with the pea shoots and edible flowers!

Cook's Note: Most markets carry hemp oil, and it is available online. If you can't find hemp oil, use extra-virgin olive oil.

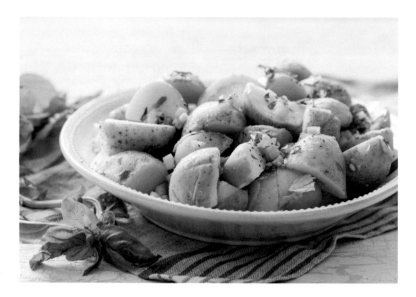

Heart Healthy Potato Salad

If you think the only way to enjoy potato salad is with lots of mayonnaise, think again, and give this potato salad a try. This recipe is low in calories, light, refreshing, and full of flavor from all the fresh herbs. Fresh herbs contain unique antioxidants, essential oils, vitamins, and many other plant-derived nutrients. Herbs help equip our body to fight against germs, toxins, and boost immunity levels.

SERVES 8

INGREDIENTS

2 pounds Yukon Gold potatoes, quartered

½ cup extra-virgin olive oil

1 tablespoon Dijon mustard

¼ cup white wine vinegar

2 tablespoons Champagne vinegar

2 tablespoons rice wine vinegar

3 tablespoons fresh lemon juice

2 tablespoons chopped Italian (flat leaf) parsley

3 tablespoons chopped fresh dill

1 tablespoon chopped fresh oregano

1 tablespoon chopped fresh mint

8 fresh basil leaves, rolled tightly and sliced into thin ribbons

1 teaspoon kosher salt and cracked black pepper

INSTRUCTIONS

1. Boil potatoes for 30 minutes or until tender. Check by inserting a paring knife through the potato. If it slides in and out easily, they are done. Drain and place in a serving bowl.

2. In a medium-sized bowl, whisk the olive oil and Dijon mustard until they're homogenized. Add the white wine vinegar, Champagne vinegar, rice wine vinegar, lemon juice, parsley, dill, oregano, mint, basil, and salt and pepper. Whisk thoroughly. Pour the vinegar mixture over the potatoes and mix gently. Season to taste, adding more salt and pepper if necessary. Serve warm, at room temperature, or cold!

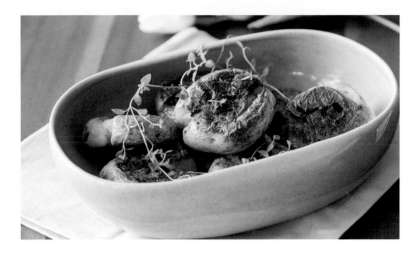

Smashed Potatoes

I sauté these potatoes with ghee. Ghee is a clarified butter that has had its milk solids browned then skimmed away from the fat, resulting in a product that combines oil's very high smoke point and butter's rich nutty flavor. The result is the delicious browned, nutty, caramel-like taste and aroma for which ghee is known.

There are numerous benefits of ghee, and some of its components have been shown to do everything from boost weight loss to improve digestion and relieve inflammation. Ghee is packed with fat soluble vitamins that can be especially crucial if you suffer from any conditions like leaky gut syndrome, IBS or Crohn's. Almost all supermarkets carry ghee.

MAKES 12 POTATOES

INGREDIENTS

12 Yukon Gold potatoes (they don't need to be precise in size but keep them small)

1 quart chicken or vegetable stock, store-bought or homemade

¼ cup Ghee (see recipe, p. 222)

4 sprigs fresh thyme, snipped

Kosher salt and cracked black pepper

½ teaspoon truffle salt, optional

INSTRUCTIONS

1. Place the potatoes into a large soup pot with the stock. Bring to a gentle boil for 45 minutes or until the potatoes are soft enough to run a knife through the center. Drain the potatoes and pat dry.

2. Using a flat-bottomed wine or olive oil bottle, gently smash the potatoes to break them open.

3. Heat a cast-iron skillet on medium-high heat for 3 minutes, add the ghee, and heat for 30 more seconds. Add the potatoes and reduce the heat to medium. Cook 4 minutes or until the bottoms turn golden and crusty.

4. Repeat with the other side. Arrange the potatoes on a platter, add the thyme, pinches of kosher salt, pepper, and truffle salt, if desired. Serve immediately.

Cook's Tip: Ghee is a healthier alternative for high heat recipes than cooking oils like canola, peanut, corn, and soybean, which are usually genetically modified and often partially hydrogenated.

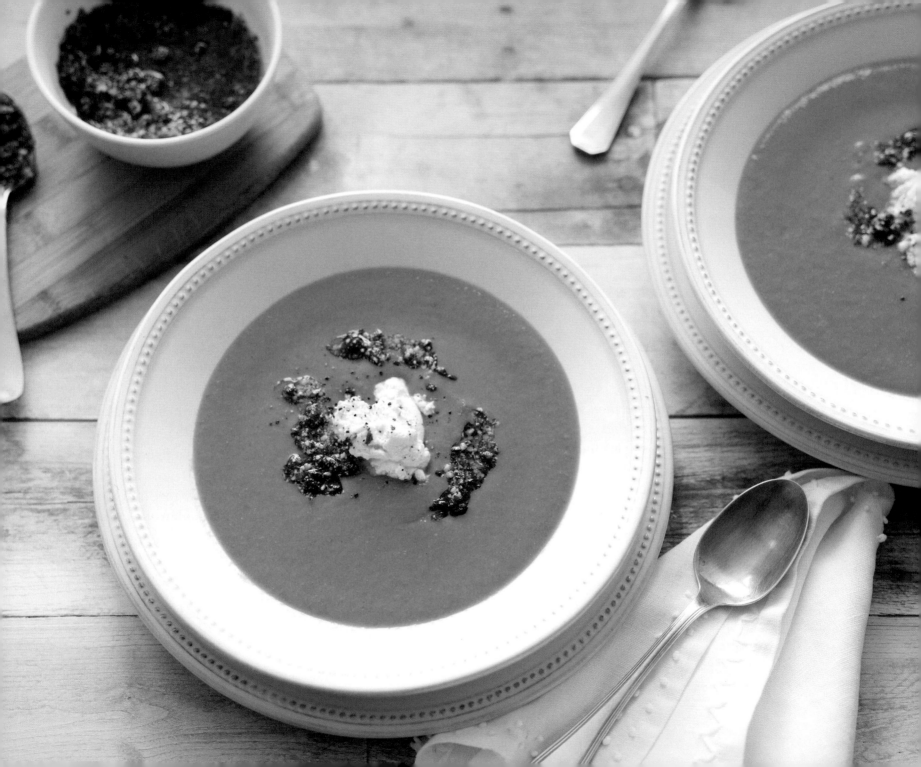

CHAPTER 5

Soup: The Ultimate Feel-Good Food

I don't know about you, but sitting down to enjoy a hot or cold bowl of soup soothes my soul! It is the ultimate feel-good meal in a bowl, and the bonus is I get most, if not all, of the nutrients I need for the day in one delicious serving.

The American Heart Association recommends adults consume 4 to 5, or more, servings of fruits and vegetables every day. Soup is a great way to get your daily intake of vegetables.

The soup recipes in this chapter are a combination of family recipes handed-down, plus today's gut, heart, and brain guidelines for healthy eating.

I don't know about you but sitting down to enjoy a hot or cold bowl of soup soothes my soul! It is the ultimate feel-good meal in a bowl, and the bonus is, I get most, if not all, of the nutrients I need for the day in one delicious serving.

The American Heart Association recommends adults consume 4 to 5, or more, servings of fruits and vegetables every day. Soup is a great way to get your daily intake of vegetables.

I particularly love creamy chilled soups, garnished with fresh herbs, nuts, and oils, such as extra-virgin olive oil, walnut, avocado, truffle, and sesame oils. These oils are healthy fats that your heart will thank you for! Soup made with beans and lean meats provide lean protein and fiber.

I chill my meat stocks overnight so the fat can congeal and rise to the top. Then I skim the fat right off without sacrificing any rich flavor.

The soup recipes in this chapter are a combination of family recipes handed down, plus today's gut, heart, and brain guidelines to healthy eating.

Choosing to make your own soup rather than using canned is a better choice because oftentimes canned soup contains the chemical BPA and is high in sodium, which is prevalent in the American diet. However, there are many great organic soups on the market that are low-sodium and chemical free. All supermarkets carry organic chicken, beef, and vegetable stock or broth.

I keep an array of stocks in my pantry at all times. They come in handy when I need to pull a meal together quickly, and they're great for making gravies and sauces. Go to the end of the chapter to get the basic recipes for homemade soups and stocks.

I like my hot soups steaming *hot*, and cold soups really *cold*!

To make sure soup stays piping hot in the bowl, I always fill the bowls with hot water and let them sit for 1 minute to take the chill off the serving bowl. You can also place the soup bowls in a preheated oven at 200°F for 10 minutes; use oven mitts to remove the soup bowls.

For chilled soups, I freeze the bowls for 20 minutes to get them super cold.

I can tomatoes in the late summer because of the abundance of summer sweet tomatoes that are available. That way I can enjoy their full-bodied goodness long into winter.

I handpicked all the soups in this chapter for their nutritional and health benefits. Delivering full flavor along with all the nutrients, antioxidants, and healing properties for your heart, mind, and body.

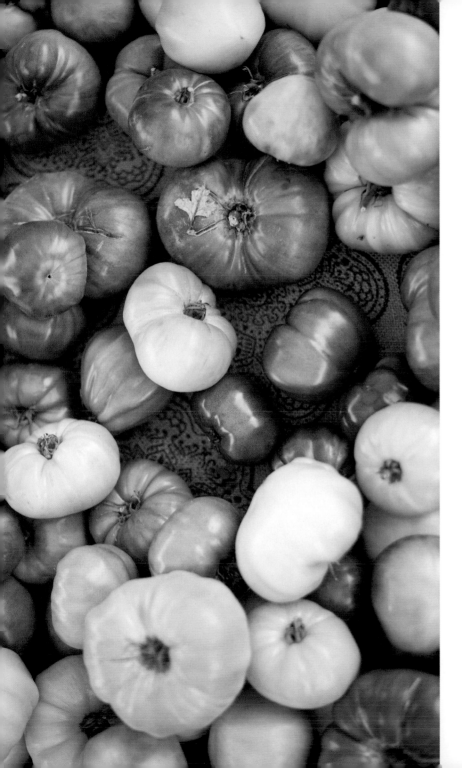

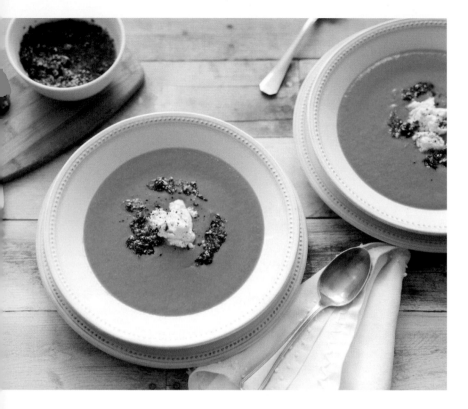

Cream of Tomato Soup with Homemade Ricotta Cheese and Arugula Pesto

As far as soups go, this is my favorite one to make, serve, and eat! It's also a very simple and quick tomato sauce for pasta, omelets, and baked dishes, such as fish or chicken. The bonus here is that it makes a delicious soup served piping hot or chilled. It's light, full of sweet tomato flavor, and is filled with the powerful antioxidant lycopene.

Lycopene improves heart health by lowering blood pressure, which helps prevent coronary heart disease, fights toxins in the blood, and helps keep your eyes healthy. Lycopene has pain-inhibiting abilities for those suffering from neuropathy, and it is good for your brain by counteracting future cell damage. It also helps keep your bones strong by helping relieve stress on the bones.

For added flavor and texture, I add homemade ricotta cheese as a garnish, and arugula pesto. You can use store-bought ricotta cheese for this recipe, but I highly recommend you make your own. It's surprisingly simple to make and the difference in the flavor and texture is like night and day.

SERVES 4 TO 6

INGREDIENTS

¼ cup, plus 6 tablespoons extra-virgin olive oil

12 scallions, white and light green parts, finely chopped

½ cup dry white wine

16 large organic Roma tomatoes, quartered

1½ teaspoons each of kosher salt and cracked black pepper

2 cups vegetable or chicken broth

Parmesan cheese, optional

Homemade Ricotta Cheese (see recipe, p. 223)

Arugula Pesto (see recipe, p. 218)

INSTRUCTIONS

1. Heat a medium saucepan on medium-high heat for one minute. Add the olive oil and scallions; reduce the heat to medium and cook 5 minutes, until the scallions release their juices. Add the wine. Cook until the liquid is reduced by more than half. Add the tomatoes, salt, and pepper. Mix well.

2. Reduce the heat to low and simmer 30 minutes. Make sure to stir a few times during cooking.

3. Place the simmered tomatoes into a food processor or blender; purée the tomato mixture for one minute.

4. Strain the tomatoes through a China cap (see Cook's Note) or medium mesh strainer to collect the seeds and skins, discard seeds and skin.

5. Pour the pureed tomatoes into a clean pot, add the broth, and simmer 20 minutes.

6. If the soup is too thick, add more chicken or vegetable stock, ¼ cup at a time, to create a smooth, creamy consistency. Taste and adjust seasoning, adding more salt if necessary.

7. Ladle the soup into heated bowls and garnish with 2 tablespoons of Homemade Ricotta Cheese and 1 tablespoon Arugula Pesto. Serve immediately.

Tip: If you are going to use this as a sauce, do not add the broth. Just mix it with your favorite pasta. You can garnish with Parmesan cheese, fresh basil, and ricotta. This soup can also be served chilled.

Cook's Note: The secret to a great fresh tomato sauce or soup is to strain it. If you don't, you will be left with a bitter-tasting sauce from the seeds and skins. I use a China cap to strain all my soups and sauces. It's shaped like a funnel and is the one tool in my kitchen I can't live without. It removes seeds and other coarse matter from soft foods. You can find China caps, or chinoise, online. If you don't have a China cap, use a strainer with holes just large enough to catch the skin and seeds. If the mesh is too tight the holes will be too small, and the tomatoes will be runny and contain too much liquid.

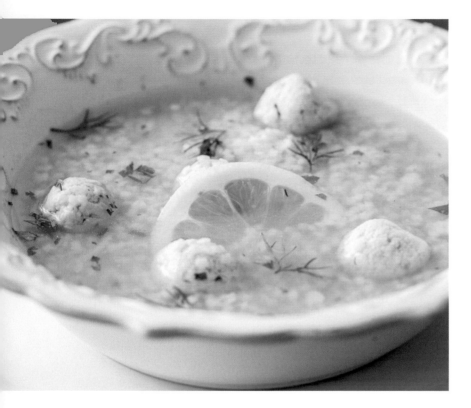

Roasted Chicken Soup with Chicken Meatballs and Baby Pastina Alla Nonna!

This dish holds a special place in our hearts around our family dinner table. It has been a staple in my family since I was a little girl, when it was made with love by my grandmother. Pastina with chicken broth and meatballs was the first solid food I remember eating as a child. I made it for my babies when they were small, and it is still their go-to meal, especially when they feel under the weather.

The fact that the broth is simmered with vegetables means it includes vitamins and nutrients, and it provides the soothing comfort that only a warm bowl of soup can provide.

The chicken meatballs are definitely a big hit with kids and adults. Everyone who has this soup for the first time comments about how light and delicious the tiny meatballs floating in their soup are, and they love the pastina.

Pastina pasta looks like teeny-tiny stars, and it's available in the pasta section in most supermarkets. If you can't find pastina, any small pasta will do. I published this recipe over ten years ago and I wanted to introduce it again; it's that special. Enjoy!

SERVES 6 TO 8

INGREDIENTS

Roasted Chicken Stock (see recipe, p. 113)

2 rotisserie chicken breasts, cut into 1-inch pieces

1 egg, slightly beaten

1 scallion, white and light green part, chopped small

3 tablespoons finely chopped fresh chives, divided

1 tablespoon finely chopped fresh Italian (flat leaf) parsley

¼ cup freshly grated Parmesan cheese, plus more for serving

¼ cup Romano cheese

⅛ teaspoon each of kosher salt and cracked black pepper

1 cup pastina or other small pasta, cooked according to package directions

INSTRUCTIONS

1. In a food processor combine the chicken, egg, scallion, 1 teaspoon chives, parsley, Parmesan and Romano cheeses, salt and pepper.

2. Pulse until the mixture comes together and forms an easy-to-roll consistency. Do not overly chop or the mixture will become pasty.

3. Shape the chicken mixture into tiny meatballs about the size of large grapes; place them on a baking sheet.

4. Using the already prepared chicken stock, bring it to a boil, lower the heat to medium-low, and add the chicken meatballs, 5 to 6 per guest. Make sure to simmer slowly; boiling too briskly will break them up.

5. Now is a good time to heat the bowls in an oven at 200F°. Make sure to *use oven mitts* to remove the bowls from the oven when you're ready to serve.

6. Add the cooked pastina to the stock with the meatballs and gently stir. Simmer 5 minutes.

7. Ladle soup into the heated bowls. Make sure everyone has at least 5 or 6 meatballs. Sprinkle each serving with more grated Parmesan cheese and the remaining chives!

8. If you are not serving immediately keep covered and bring up to a gentle boil on medium high heat for 8 to 10 minutes before serving.

9. This soup will keep in the refrigerator in an airtight container for 2 days. You can freeze the chicken meatballs for up to 6 months.

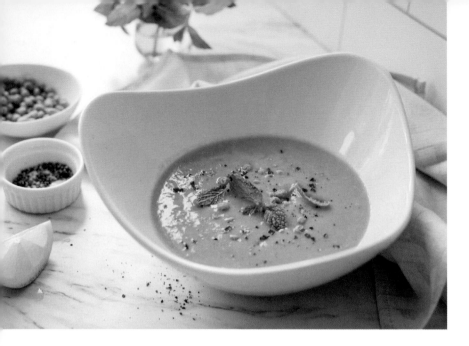

English Spring Garden Pea Soup

Who knew that this teeny-tiny green orb is considered one of the healthiest foods on the planet? Green peas are filled with most of the daily nutrients a body requires to stay healthy. In warmer weather, I serve this soup cold in shot glasses as a teaser appetizer, or in a chilled bowl with a delicate butter lettuce salad on the side. It is also amazing piping hot in the cold winter months! I add crispy shallots over the top, a drizzle of walnut oil, and a pinch of cayenne! Warms the heart and tummy!

Green peas are a rich source of calcium, iron, copper, zinc, and vitamin K, for blood coagulation, and provide nearly a quarter of the daily need for thiamin, vitamin A, and folate.

This soup takes 15 minutes to make (unless shelling fresh peas). I can't wait for spring when the peas are sweet and tender. I always have organic frozen peas in my freezer when fresh peas are not available.

SERVES 6

INGREDIENTS

2 cups chicken or vegetable stock, store-bought or homemade

3 pounds (about 3½ cups) fresh English peas, shelled, or a 1 pound bag frozen petite peas

½ teaspoon kosher salt

6 teaspoons of finely chopped fresh chives

10 fresh mint leaves, torn into small pieces

6 teaspoons walnut oil

6 teaspoons pistachio nuts

A pinch of large flake sea salt

INSTRUCTIONS

1. In a large saucepan, bring the stock to a boil. Add the peas and cook 6 minutes or until the peas are tender. If you're using frozen peas boil 2 to 3 minutes.

2. Pour the peas into a blender, add salt and process for 1 minute, until the mixture is smooth and creamy.

3. Cover and chill in the refrigerator for 3 hours. Fifteen minutes before serving place the soup and the bowls in the freezer to get them extra chilled!

4. Garnish each serving with 1 teaspoon of chives, some mint leaves, 1 teaspoon walnut oil, 1 teaspoon of pistachio, and sea salt.

Basic Chicken Soup

One of the most loved "feel-good" foods, just about everyone has a personal spin on a chicken soup recipe. Rarely have such simple ingredients created so much comfort. This version has classic flavors and is oh-so soothing, especially if you feel a cold or flu coming on, but you can enjoy it anytime. There's no need to use a separate stock; the vegetables and meat form their own satisfying broth. The broth is filled with nutrients that will help boost your immune system and reduce inflammation.

MAKES 2½ QUARTS

INGREDIENTS

3 quarts water

1 tablespoon kosher salt

6 peppercorns

1 (5-pound) raw organic chicken

2 medium yellow onions, skins on, quartered

6 scallions, white and green parts, chopped

4 celery ribs with tops, chopped

4 large carrots, peeled and chopped

½ bunch Italian (flat leaf) parsley

INSTRUCTIONS

1. Add the water, salt, peppercorns, chicken, onions, scallions, celery, carrots, and parsley to a large stockpot. Bring to a rapid boil on high heat. Reduce the heat to a bubbling simmer and partially cover with a lid; simmer 90 minutes. Stir every 30 minutes.

2. Remove the chicken from the pot and place it into a separate bowl to cool. Remove the meat from the bones, cover and set aside.

3. Strain the soup through a mesh strainer. Discard chicken bones and vegetables. Correct seasoning by adding more salt if necessary.

4. Refrigerate the soup overnight. The fat will rise to the top and you can easily remove it using a spoon.

Cook's Note: Use the extra chicken meat for sandwiches, chicken salad, enchiladas, tacos, chicken meatballs for soup, or cut into chunks to enjoy in this soup.

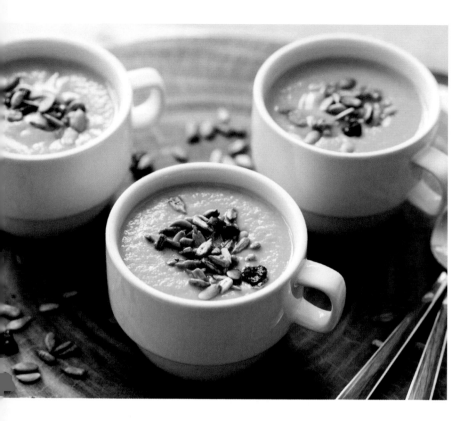

Curry Carrot Green Apple Soup with Balsamic Glaze

Curry powder is a spice mix that has numerous health benefits. Listen to this: it helps protects your heart against disease and will ease pain and inflammation in the body. It reduces Alzheimer's disease symptoms, boosts bone health, and protects the immune system from bacterial infections.

The carrots in this soup are rich in vitamin A, which benefits eye health, and vitamins C, K, B as well as folate, potassium, iron, copper, and manganese. It improves blood pressure, helps the skin, and has anti-aging properties.

The apples are rich in vitamins A, B, C, and folic acid. Apples aid in digestion, are rich in fiber, improve intestinal health, aid in respiratory issues, and help prevent heart disease—plus they are simply delicious!

I serve this soup often to my family and guests. I was honored to find out that this soup was chosen to be served at a luncheon at City of Hope Hospital for a recent seminar on cancer research.

SERVES 4 TO 6

INGREDIENTS

¼ cup extra-virgin olive oil

1 large yellow onion, peeled, cut in half and sliced thin

6 scallions, white and light green parts, coarsely chopped

2 tablespoons dry sherry

6 medium carrots, peeled and chopped into chunks

1 large green apple, peeled, cored, and chopped into chunks

2 tablespoons curry powder

1½ quarts vegetable or chicken broth

2 teaspoons each kosher salt and cracked black pepper

4 to 6 sprigs of fresh dill, coarsely chopped

6 teaspoons walnut oil

¼ cup sunflower seeds

¼ cup pumpkin seeds

½ cup Toasted Walnuts, chopped (see recipe, p. 221)

Pinch of Cayenne pepper

Balsamic Glaze, store-bought or homemade
　　(see recipe, p. 212)

INSTRUCTIONS

1. Heat a large soup pot on medium-high heat for 30 seconds. Add the olive oil, onion, and scallions; sauté 6 to 8 minutes or until the veggies release their juices and the onion is translucent.

2. Add the sherry, carrots, apple, and curry powder; mix well. Stir for 1 minute to "wake up" the flavor of the curry.

3. Add the stock, salt, and black pepper. Lower the heat to medium. Cover the soup pot and bring to a gentle, low boil for 30 minutes.

4. Working in batches, ladle the soup into a blender and process for 1 minute for a smooth and creamy consistency. Transfer the processed soup to another bowl while you finish blending the remaining soup.

5. Pour the processed soup into a clean soup pot and reheat 8 to 10 minutes on medium heat. Ladle into the preheated bowls.

6. Garnish each serving with dill. Drizzle 1 teaspoon of walnut oil over each serving. Sprinkle some sunflower and pumpkin seeds and toasted walnuts on top.

7. Finish with a pinch of cayenne pepper and a drizzle of the Balsamic Glaze.

Cook's Note: This is perfect as a summer soup too! Serve it chilled and pair it with a green garden salad.

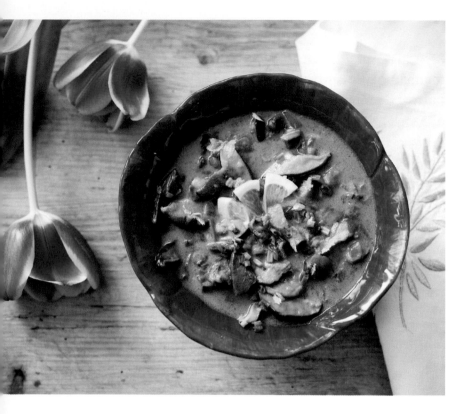

Five Mushroom Medley

Mushroom lovers rejoice: this is the best mushroom soup I've ever made. I love mushrooms and one of my favorite ways to prepare them is to sauté a variety to make this savory soup, which has a surprisingly light and delicate broth. I use several varieties of mushrooms to enhance the flavor: Portobello, shiitake, cremini, plus white and brown buttons—five different kinds of mushrooms, each with their own healing properties.

Mushrooms are full of gut-healing and heart-smart properties, so always keep in mind the importance of gut health. Mushrooms also help the body store energy from foods and help form red blood cells. Mushrooms are a rich source of a number of B vitamins, which appear to be important for a healthy brain. Mushrooms are the only vegan source of non-fortified vitamin D. Dairy products are normally a good food source of vitamin D, but vegans do not consume any animal products, so mushrooms offer an alternative source of this important vitamin.

SERVES 4 TO 6

INGREDIENTS

¼ cup extra-virgin olive oil

1 large white onion, peeled and diced small

3 scallions, white and light green parts, finely chopped

3 cloves garlic, finely chopped

1 (10-ounce) package *each* of sliced white button, cremini, and brown button mushrooms

2 large Portobello mushrooms, chopped small

10 shiitake mushrooms, stems removed, caps thinly sliced

1 teaspoons each kosher salt and cracked black pepper

3 tablespoons dry sherry

1 cup organic vegetable broth

1 cup organic canned Thai coconut milk

1 bay leaf

1 tablespoon regular or gluten-free soy sauce

4 to 6 tablespoons regular or vegan sour cream

3 tablespoons chives, finely chopped

2 tablespoons finely chopped fresh Italian (flat leaf) parsley

4 to 6 sprigs fresh thyme

Zest from one lemon

Pinch of cayenne pepper

INSTRUCTIONS

1. In a large stockpot over medium-high heat, add the olive oil and heat 30 seconds. Add the onion and scallions; sauté 6 minutes until the onion becomes translucent. Add the garlic and sauté 2 minutes.

2. Add the white button, cremini, brown button, Portobello, and shiitake mushrooms and the salt and pepper. Cook 5 to 8 minutes, uncovered. A substantial amount of liquid will be released by the mushrooms; cook until the liquid is reduced and mushrooms start to sizzle. Add the sherry and stir.

3. Add the broth, coconut milk, bay leaf, and soy sauce. Bring to a boil on high heat. Lower the heat and gently simmer 15 minutes until the soup starts to thicken, stirring occasionally. Taste the soup and season as desired, adding more salt and pepper if necessary.

4. Ladle into preheated bowls and garnish each serving with 1 tablespoon sour cream, some chopped chives, parsley, several thyme leaves pulled from the sprigs, lemon zest, and a pinch of cayenne pepper. Lay the thyme sprigs over the soup to serve.

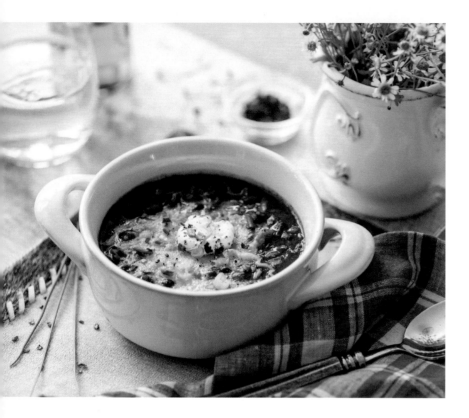

Protein-Packed Black Bean Soup

We eat a variety of beans in our home. I have one child who is a vegan, another who is a vegetarian, and one who cannot digest animal protein—so beans it is, every time they come over. Vegetarians and individuals who seldom eat meat, poultry, or fish, like me, can count on beans as an alternate choice. When you combine beans with brown rice it is a "complete protein," making vegetarians everywhere very happy.

Black beans are packed with nutrients that affect our bodies in many ways. They are high in fiber and protein, and full of vitamins and minerals. Beans are a great way for you to get protein, they have a low glycemic index, and contain a blend of complex carbohydrates and protein. Because of this, beans are digested slowly, which helps keep blood glucose stable and may help curtail fatigue and irritability. Scientists recommend that adults consume 3 cups of beans per week to promote health and reduce the risk of chronic diseases, like cancer, because of their abundance of antioxidants.

Dietary Guidelines indicate we should be eating more plant proteins. A half-cup of beans provides 7 grams of protein, which is the same amount as in 1 ounce of chicken, meat, or fish.

SERVES 4 TO 6

INGREDIENTS

¼ cup extra-virgin olive oil, plus more for drizzling

1 large yellow onion, peeled and diced

2 tablespoons diced shallots

3 cloves garlic, minced

1 small red or yellow bell pepper, seeded and diced

1 tablespoon ground cumin

1 tablespoon ground coriander

2 tablespoons ground chili powder

1 tablespoon onion powder

1 tablespoon garlic powder

1 teaspoon kosher salt

1 quart vegetable broth, plus more to thin the soup
(if needed)

3 (15-ounce) cans black beans, 1 can rinsed and drained

2 jalapeños with seeds, finely chopped

1 cup coarsely chopped cilantro

2 cups aged sharp regular or vegan Cheddar cheese, grated

½ cup regular or vegan sour cream

½ cup diced red onion

4 sprigs thyme, leaves stripped off

INSTRUCTIONS

1. Heat a large soup pot on medium-high heat for 30 seconds. Add the olive oil, onion, shallots, and garlic. Sauté 8 minutes.

2. Add the bell pepper, cumin, coriander, chili powder, onion powder, garlic powder, and salt. Sauté 1 minute. Add the broth and the 2 cans of undrained black beans.

3. Lower the heat and simmer 60 minutes, checking every 15 minutes to make sure that the beans are not sticking to the sides and bottom of the pan. If the soup is too thick just add more vegetable broth, ½ cup at a time, to thin.

4. Ten minutes before serving, turn the heat to medium. Add the can of rinsed black beans to the pot and heat through, 5 minutes on medium heat.

5. Ladle into heated bowls and garnish each serving with jalapeño, as much as you like, some cilantro, a helping of cheddar cheese, a dollop of sour cream, 1 tablespoon red onions, a drizzle of olive oil, and a pinch of thyme leaves.

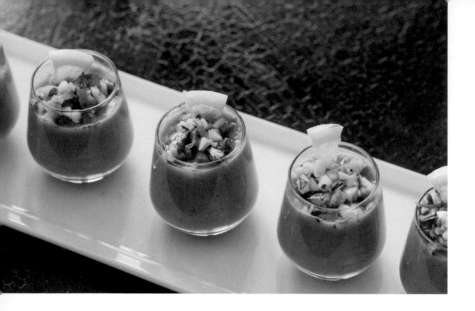

Gazpacho with Habanero Cucumber Pineapple Salsa!

The hot, humid, sweet summer months are the perfect time to enjoy gazpacho, when vine-ripened tomatoes are at their peak of flavor. It's a beautiful blend of tomatoes, cucumber, sweet bell peppers, onions, fresh garden herbs, and other summer veggies and fruits. Gazpacho tastes even better the next day, after all the wonderful flavors have had a chance to sit overnight.

This cold soup is filled with everything your body needs for nutrients; the vitamins and antioxidants keep your body healthy. You get the extra benefits of the fruits and veggies because you are eating them raw. Make the Habanero Pineapple Salsa first so the flavors have time to meld. Enjoy with a warm crusty loaf of bread!

GAZPACHO

SERVES 6

INGREDIENTS

3 thick slices sourdough bread, crusts removed
    and torn into pieces

½ cup water

12 medium-sized ripe Roma tomatoes

1 cup chopped red onion

½ medium red bell pepper, seeded and cut into chunks

1 large cucumber, peeled and seeded; cut into chunks

2 teaspoons garlic powder

3 tablespoons extra-virgin olive oil plus more for garnish

3 tablespoons sherry wine vinegar

2 tablespoons rice wine vinegar

3 scallions, white and light green parts, coarsely chopped

2 teaspoons each of kosher salt and cracked black pepper

1 cup Croutons (see recipe, p. 222)

Large flake sea salt or coarse salt

Crushed red pepper

2 limes cut into wedges

INSTRUCTIONS

1. Place the bread in a small bowl, add the water, and soak 5 minutes. Squeeze all the water out and place the soaked bread in a large bowl.

2. Bring 2 quarts of water to a boil in a medium soup pot. With a paring knife, cut an "X" on the tops or sides of the tomatoes. Place 6 tomatoes in the boiling water for 30 to 45 seconds. Remove each with slotted spoon and place into a bowl of cool water. Repeat the process with the remaining tomatoes. Remove the skins; discard.

3. Slice the tomatoes in half from top to bottom, remove the seeds, and discard. Chop the tomatoes into small pieces and add them to the bowl with the bread.

4. Add the onion, bell pepper, chopped cucumber, garlic powder, olive oil, both vinegars, scallions, salt, and pepper. Mix well. Cover with plastic wrap and place the bowl on a counter for 1 hour to allow the flavors to meld.

5. Pour the tomato mixture into a blender and process 3 minutes until it's smooth. Season by adding more salt if necessary. Cover tightly with plastic wrap and refrigerate 4 hours before serving.

6. It can be made the day before, which I prefer. It gives more time for all the wonderful flavors to come together.

7. When you're ready to serve, freeze the serving bowls about 30 minutes to get them super chilled.

8. For each serving, scoop one to two ladlesful of soup into the chilled bowls, and garnish with 1 to 2 tablespoons pineapple salsa and the croutons.

9. Drizzle 2 teaspoons extra-virgin olive oil over each bowl, and add a pinch of finishing salt and a pinch of crushed red pepper. Serve with a lime wedge!

HABAÑERO PINEAPPLE SALSA

YIELD 2½ CUPS

INGREDIENTS

2 cups pineapple, diced

½ cup cucumber, skinned, seeded, and diced

½ mango, diced

2 scallions, white and light green part, finely chopped

2 tablespoons fresh lemon juice

2 tablespoons fresh lime juice

2 tablespoons rice wine vinegar

½ teaspoon each kosher salt and cracked black pepper

2 tablespoons finely chopped cilantro

1 tablespoon Italian (flat leaf) parsley, finely chopped

3 tablespoons extra-virgin olive oil

1 small habañero chile pepper with seeds, finely chopped (see Cook's Note)

INSTRUCTIONS

Place the pineapple, cucumber, mango, scallions, lemon juice, lime juice, rice wine vinegar, salt, pepper, cilantro, parsley, olive oil, and chile pepper into a glass bowl. Mix well and cover with plastic wrap. Refrigerate for 2 hours.

Cook's Note: Habañero chile peppers are one of the hottest peppers, so you can substitute jalapeño peppers or eliminate the peppers all together. But I have to say, the little bit of heat gives this gazpacho a bit of a kick!

Tip: The salsa can be made the night before and refrigerated. It will keep in the refrigerator in a tightly sealed glass jar for 2 days.

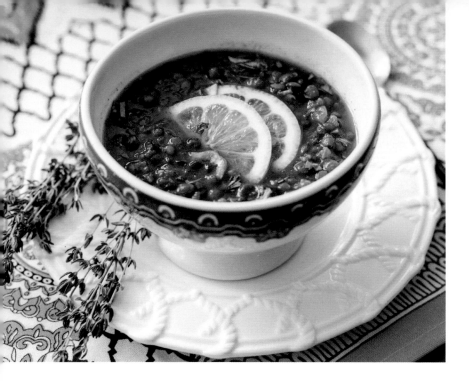

South African Red Lentil Soup with Spiced Oil

This recipe hails from South Africa, where I had the honor to attend the opening of Oprah's school, The Leadership Academy for Girls. On the menu was a soup made with red lentils and African spices. It was so delicious that I went right up to the cook who was serving the last portions from a heavy, cast-iron skillet, and simply asked him if he would share the recipe. He smiled at me and said yes. Lucky me!

I am sharing this lentil soup recipe not only because it is delicious, but also because of the many health benefits of lentils. Lentils have components that are necessary for gut health. Lentils help lower cholesterol and are great for heart and digestive health. They stabilize blood sugar, help increase energy, and are a great source of protein.

I buy the best quality spices in small packets from the health food store, because smaller portions preserve the spices and they are full of potent flavor.

My recipe includes Spiced Oil. Drizzle it on the soup—if you like an extra kick!

SERVES 4 TO 6

INGREDIENTS

3 tablespoons extra-virgin olive oil
1 large yellow onion, finely chopped
2 garlic cloves peeled and minced
1 teaspoon each salt and pepper
1 tablespoon ground cumin
2 teaspoons ground coriander
¼ teaspoon ground ginger
¼ teaspoon ground cinnamon
½ teaspoon cayenne
1 tablespoon tomato paste
2 quarts chicken or vegetable broth, divided
2 cups water
1½ cups (10.5 ounces) red lentils
2 tablespoons lemon juice
¼ cup coarsely chopped cilantro
2 lemons, one thinly sliced, one cut into 8 wedges

INSTRUCTIONS

1. In a soup pot on medium heat add the onion and olive oil and cook 8 minutes, stirring occasionally, until the onion has softened. Add the garlic, salt, and pepper; cook 1 minute.

2. Add the cumin, coriander, ginger, cinnamon, cayenne, and tomato paste. Mix well. Turn the heat to low and cook 1 minute, stirring constantly.

3. Pour in 1½ quarts of chicken or vegetable broth and bring to a boil. Turn the heat to low and simmer 15 minutes.

4. Add the lentils and bring to boil, then turn the heat to low.

5. Simmer, stirring occasionally, until lentils are soft, approximately 30 minutes or a bit more. Test to see if the lentils are cooked through; they should be soft but not mushy. If you see the soup is too thick add more broth, ½ cup at a time.

6. Stir in the lemon juice and season, adding a pinch more salt if needed.

7. Ladle the soup into individual heated bowls. Drizzle each portion with 2 teaspoons or more of the spiced oil, depending on how spicy you like it. Sprinkle with the cilantro, garnish with a sliced lemon, and serve with a lemon wedge on the side.

Tip: This soup can be refrigerated for up to 3 days. Thin the soup with chicken or vegetable broth when reheating.

SPICED OIL

INGREDIENTS

⅓ cup extra-virgin olive oil

1 small clove garlic, smashed

2 teaspoons dried mint, crumbled

1 teaspoon paprika

2 teaspoons crushed red pepper

¼ cup chopped fresh cilantro

INSTRUCTIONS

Combine the olive oil, garlic, mint, paprika, crushed red pepper, and cilantro into a Mason jar or other small glass container with a lid. Shake well and set aside at room temperature until you're ready to use it.

Cook's Note: Any leftover Spiced Oil can be saved to drizzle over omelets, eggs, avocado toast, creamy soups, grilled fish, or grilled veggies!

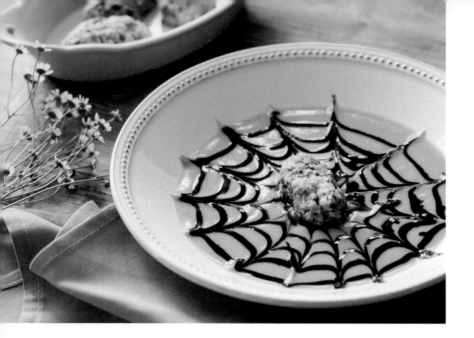

Roasted Butternut Squash Soup with Balsamic Surprise!

I love making this velvety soup in the fall. It's filling and satisfying, and my home smells like the holidays because of all the simmering spices. My kids remember how I insisted on Halloween that they first have a warm bowl of soup before we went "trick or treating."

Butternut squash is low in fat and rich in dietary fiber, making it a heart-friendly choice. It provides significant amounts of potassium, important for bone health. It has an abundance of carotenoids, shown to protect against heart disease. Because of its high abundance of antioxidants, squash helps reduce risk of inflammation-related disorders, such as rheumatoid arthritis and asthma.

4 TO 6 SERVINGS

INGREDIENTS

1 (3-pound) butternut squash

¼ cup extra-virgin olive oil, plus 1 tablespoon

2 medium onions, peeled and thinly sliced

5 scallions, white and light green parts, coarsely chopped

1 tablespoon dry sherry

1½ teaspoons each of kosher salt and cracked black pepper

1 teaspoon ground cinnamon

Pinch of ground cloves

½ teaspoon grated nutmeg

1 quart chicken or vegetable broth

4 ounces non- or low-fat cream cheese at room temperature, cut into pieces

6 to 8 tablespoons low-fat or vegan sour cream

1 jalapeño with seeds, finely diced

2 tablespoons pomegranate seeds

Pinch of cayenne pepper

½ teaspoon per serving truffle oil, extra-virgin olive oil, or walnut oil, for garnish

Balsamic Glaze (see recipe, p. 212)

INSTRUCTIONS

1. Preheat the oven to 350F°.

2. Place the squash on a rimmed baking sheet. Drizzle with 1 tablespoon olive oil; coat the whole squash. Bake 45 minutes or until you can insert a knife through the squash smoothly. Remove and allow it to cool 20 minutes. Using a knife, open the squash to remove the seeds; discard the seeds. Scrape out the flesh; discard the rind.

3. Heat a large soup pot on medium high heat for 1 minute. Add ¼ cup olive oil and heat for 30 seconds. Add the onion and scallions; cook 5 to 8 minutes. Add the sherry, baked squash, salt, pepper, cinnamon, cloves, and nutmeg. Mix well. Add the broth and bring it to a boil. Lower the heat and simmer 30 minutes.

4. Pour 3 cups of the soup into a blender and add the cream cheese. Blend for 1 minute and pour into a clean stockpot. Blend the remaining squash, add to the stockpot and mix together well. Taste and adjust the seasoning by adding more salt and pepper if necessary.

VEGETABLE QUENELLE

A quenelle is an oval-shaped dumpling made either with meat or vegetables. I make mine using vegetables. You can make them beforehand and refrigerate until ready to use.

MAKES 6 TO 8

INGREDIENTS

4 tablespoons extra-virgin olive oil

2 tablespoons minced shallots

2 small zucchini, finely chopped

¼ cup carrots, peeled and finely chopped

¼ teaspoon kosher salt

1 tablespoon fresh lemon juice

3 tablespoons freshly grated Parmesan cheese

3 tablespoons regular or gluten-free breadcrumbs

1 tablespoon finely chopped Italian (flat leaf) parsley

2 teaspoons chives, finely chopped

INSTRUCTIONS

1. Preheat the oven to 200F°.

2. Heat a cast-iron skillet or heavy-bottomed skillet for 1 minute on medium-high heat. Add the olive oil and swirl to coat the bottom of the pan. Reduce the heat to medium, add the shallots, and cook 2 minutes or until they start to caramelize.

3. Add the zucchini, carrots, and salt. Cook until almost all of the liquid that's released from the zucchini has cooked down and you can hear a sizzle.

4. Pour the zucchini mixture into a bowl and cool 15 minutes. Add the lemon juice, Parmesan cheese, breadcrumbs, parsley, and chives. Mix well.

5. To shape into quenelles, take two teaspoons and fill one with a scoop of the zucchini mixture. Roll the mix back and forth between the two spoons until you have a solid oval shape. It may take 4 to 5 passes before you have the perfect shape. Place each quenelle gently on a plate. Cover them lightly with foil, making sure the foil doesn't touch the quenelles. Keep them warm in the preheated oven until you're ready to serve. Enjoy!

Tip: Make the spider web when you are ready to serve the soup. Ladle a serving into warmed soup bowls. Make 4 circles with the Balsamic Glaze, starting from the widest part of the bowl, working your way into the center. To make the design for the spider web, take the point of a knife, place it in the middle of the smallest circle, and drag it towards the rim of the plate. Repeat this process until you have formed a spider web. Place the quenelle in the middle.

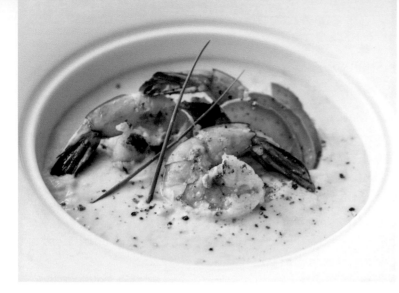

Chilled Avocado Soup
with Spicy Shrimp

Avocados are incredibly nutritious: they contain more potassium than bananas, and are loaded with heart-healthy monounsaturated fatty acids and fiber. This is one of my favorite recipes for avocado soup, and the grilled shrimp puts it over the top!

SERVES 4 TO 5

INGREDIENTS

1 cup buttermilk

3 ripe avocados, peeled and pitted

⅓ cup full-fat Greek yogurt, plain

2 tablespoons diced white onion

1 scallion, white and light green part, chopped

1 tablespoon jalapeño with seeds, finely chopped

½ cup fresh lime juice, divided

2 cups vegetable stock

8 large raw shrimp, peeled and deveined

½ teaspoon chili powder

⅛ teaspoon cayenne pepper

1 teaspoon onion powder

1 teaspoon garlic powder

2 teaspoon kosher salt, divided

1 teaspoon cracked black pepper

3 tablespoons extra-virgin olive oil

1 lime, cut into wedges

Spicy Mango Salsa (see recipe, p. 223)

INSTRUCTIONS

1. In a blender, combine the buttermilk, avocados, yogurt, onion, scallion, jalapeño, 1 teaspoon of the salt, ¼ cup of the lime juice, and stock. Blend for 1 minute. If the soup is too thick, add a bit more stock until it has the consistancy of a creamy soup. Refrigerate 2 hours.

2. In a small bowl whisk the chili powder, cayenne pepper, onion powder, garlic powder, remaining 1 teaspoon of salt, pepper, olive oil, and remaining ¼ cup of lime juice. Pour over the shrimp. Cover and marinate in the refrigerator for 1 hour.

3. About 30 minutes before serving, preheat the oven to 450F°. Remove the shrimp from the refrigerator and lay them on a baking sheet. Roast 12 minutes.

4. To serve, top each bowl with 2 to 3 shrimp, 1 tablespoon Mango Salsa, and a lime wedge.

Roasted Chicken Stock

I love the full-bodied flavor of roasted chicken stock and using the bones from an already roasted chicken gives the stock a deep, rich chicken flavor. You can use it for many dishes, including gravies, braising liquid, risotto, quinoa, pasta, and even to boil potatoes. The stock will keep up to 3 days in the refrigerator and 6 months in the freezer.

MAKES 2 QUARTS

INGREDIENTS

1 (4- to 5-pound) roasted chicken
2 yellow onions, skins on, quartered
6 scallions, chopped in half
5 garlic cloves, skins on, smashed
½ bunch Italian (flat leaf) parsley
4 large carrots, peeled and chopped
8 celery ribs with tops, chopped
1 tablespoon kosher salt
6 peppercorns
1 tablespoon ground cumin

INSTRUCTIONS

1. Separate the meat from the skin and bones of the chicken. Place the bones and skin in a stockpot and add the onions, scallions, garlic, parsley, carrots, celery, salt, peppercorns, and cumin. Cover with water by 2 inches.

2. On high heat bring the stock to a rolling boil, then turn the heat down to a low boil for 1 hour.

3. Remove from heat to cool for an hour before you strain the stock.

4. Pour strained stock into glass jars or other containers. Store in the refrigerator overnight. The fat will rise to the top and congeal; skim off the fat before serving.

Cook's Note: Place the chicken meat into a container and refrigerate it until you're ready to use it. You can use the chicken meat for sandwiches, chicken salad, enchiladas, and tacos or cut into pieces to add back into the soup.

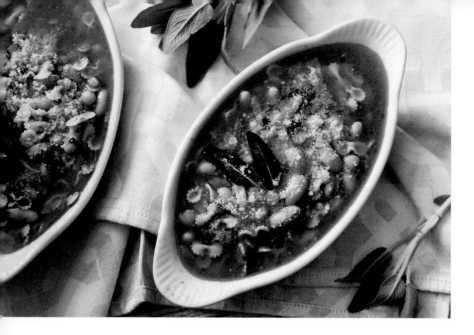

Pasta Fagioli

This recipe for Pasta Fagioli is from the northern region in Italy where my grandmother was born. It's served with a drizzle of extra-virgin olive oil, freshly grated Parmesan cheese, warm out-of-the-oven crusty Italian bread, along with a beautiful bottle of red or white wine! (Yes, I eat the bread when in Italy; I can't help it!) There is something so special about sitting around the family table enjoying music, laughter, conversation, wine, and great food.

I eat and serve beans with almost every meal—in salads, whip them to spread on rice cakes, mix them with rice and pastas, and in soups. This is an easy recipe to prepare and will be ready to serve in less than an hour. When I don't have time to soak and boil fresh beans, I use canned organic cannellini or white navy beans.

Beans are "heart healthy" and contain an abundance of soluble fiber, which can lower cholesterol and triglyceride levels. They are loaded with nutrients—vitamin B, calcium, potassium, folate, and are a rich source of protein. They are also low in fat, balance blood sugar, and the fiber helps you feel fuller, longer. Adding rice to beans can turn an incomplete protein into a complete one. Beans are filled with antioxidants and help reduce risk of cancer and diabetes.

SERVES 4 TO 6

INGREDIENTS

⅓ cup extra-virgin olive oil

1 large onion, peeled and finely chopped

3 garlic cloves, peeled and finely chopped

½ cup white wine

2 cups canned crushed tomatoes in purée

1 teaspoon each kosher salt and cracked black pepper

¼ teaspoon crushed red pepper

1½ cups small pasta (such as shells, farfalle, or your favorite kind)

3 cups chicken or vegetable broth

2 (15-ounce) cans cannellini beans, with juice

Freshly grated Parmesan or Romano cheese

Fresh thyme sprigs

Crushed red pepper, optional

8 to 10 teaspoons Arugula Pesto, divided (see recipe, p. 218)

Balsamic Glaze (see recipe, p. 212)

Fried Sage Leaves (see recipe, opposite)

INSTRUCTIONS

1. In a medium-sized soup pot, heat the olive oil on medium high heat for 30 seconds. Add the onion; sauté 5 minutes to release their natural juices. Add the garlic; sauté 2 minutes.

2. Add the wine and cook, reducing the liquid by half. Add the tomatoes, salt, pepper, and crushed red pepper. Simmer on low heat for 30 minutes.

3. While the sauce is simmering cook the pasta according to package directions. Rinse in cool water and drain.

4. When the sauce is done, add the broth and beans. Simmer 15 minutes on medium heat. Add the pasta and heat 5 more minutes until the soup gets really hot.

5. Ladle into preheated bowls, garnish with Parmesan cheese, and 2 teaspoons of Arugula Pesto drizzled over each serving. Drizzle with the Balsamic Glaze; add two fried sage leaves and crushed red pepper. Serve immediately!

Cook's Note: If the soup is too thick, just add more broth, ¼ cup at a time. This soup should be smooth and creamy, not thick and sticky!

FRIED SAGE LEAVES

INGREDIENTS

8 sage leaves
3 tablespoons extra-virgin olive oil

INSTRUCTIONS

In a small frying pan, heat 3 tablespoons extra-virgin olive oil on high heat for 1 minute. Add 8 sage leaves and fry until crisp. Drain them on paper towels until you're ready to use.

The Health Benefits of Gut-Healing Bone Broth

Bone broth is a rich infusion of beef, chicken, bison, lamb, or fish stocks. Research shows that drinking bone broth can boost one's immune system and fight inflammation. Why is inflammation dangerous? Inflammation causes distress in the body, leaving it vulnerable to a wide variety of diseases, such as Alzheimer's, cancer, heart disease, diabetes, and stroke.

Scientists have discovered that your health depends on the health of your intestinal tract. Basically, any disease of the body starts with gut health, or should I say, the lack thereof. Many articles have been written on the importance of the gut-healing properties of bone broth.

Because of its high collagen content, bone broth helps digestion, alleviates the symptoms of allergies, improves immune and brain health, supports your joints, hair, skin, nails, and does so much more. It is also high in calcium, magnesium, and phosphorus, making it a must for bone health. Research is making a connection to Alzheimer's, rheumatoid arthritis, inflammatory bowel disease, obesity, osteoporosis, and depression.

I started making bone broth several months ago because I began to have tummy issues and my joints started to hurt. It totally freaked me out. Of course, I scoured the internet to find a solution to my tummy problems. That's when I discovered the miracle of drinking bone broth. I started drinking a cup a day, and I noticed a difference in my stomach almost right away. Within a few weeks, the pain in my joints started to dissipate and my digestion improved.

The stock needs to simmer over very low heat for at least 12 hours. (Usually 24 hours is the minimum but who has the time for that? Plus, it needs to simmer throughout the night and I'm not comfortable leaving my gas range on all night.) If you are thinking, Wow! 12 hours is a long time, it is. You need to give the bone marrow, collagen, and amino acids time to soak into the stock.

Simmering low and slow for many hours helps to pull out all the necessary nutrients. Roasting the bones for 30 minutes with the vegetables first brings out the rich, smooth flavor of beef, and will give a rich, deep, beefy flavor to the broth.

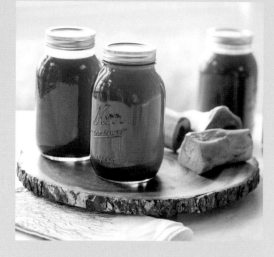

I make bone broth once a week and sip it throughout the day. I make sure to drink at least one 8-ounce glass every single day. I also serve ½ cup to my family before dinner—piping hot like a warm hug and cozy appetizer that makes your tummy feel great! I wholeheartedly encourage you to start drinking bone broth today.

Bone broth can be used to make soups, stews, chili, gravies, sauces, and reductions. If anyone in my family is ill or has a tummy ache, I serve them bone broth. It's easy to digest and helps shorten the duration of the illness.

Beef Bone Broth

MAKES 2 QUARTS

INGREDIENTS

¼ cup extra-virgin olive oil

3 pounds organic grass-fed beef bones, cut into 4-inch pieces

2 pounds organic grass-fed oxtails

2 large onions, skins on, quartered

12 scallions, white and light green parts, coarsely chopped

8 carrots, scrubbed and coarsely chopped

8 celery ribs with tops, coarsely chopped

1 head garlic, cut in half

5 quarts water (approximately)

1 bunch fresh Italian (flat leaf) parsley

1 tablespoon kosher salt

2 tablespoons apple cider vinegar

INSTRUCTIONS

1. Preheat the oven to 400°F.

2. In a large roasting pan, place the olive oil, beef bones, oxtails, onions, scallions, carrots, celery, and garlic. Sprinkle with salt and roast for 30 minutes, turning at least once.

3. Place the roasted vegetables and bones into a large stockpot. Cover with water by at least 2 inches over the bones; add the parsley, salt, and vinegar.

4. Mix well and bring to a rapid boil. Reduce the heat to super low (if you're using a gas range, do not let the flame extinguish). Cover the stockpot with a lid and simmer gently for 12 hours.

5. Check periodically. Remove any foam or sediments that rise to top. Turn off the heat and cool the broth for 1 hour.

6. Strain the bone broth using a mesh strainer. Use a funnel to pour the broth into a large wide-mouth Mason jar, leaving a good inch from the top. Seal tightly.

7. Refrigerate overnight. As the broth cools, the fat will rise to the top and congeal. Skim all the fat off and discard. Store beef broth in the refrigerator for up to 5 days.

Cook's Note: Get the bones from your butcher to make bone broth. Make sure they are from organic grass-fed cattle, raised with no additives or hormones.

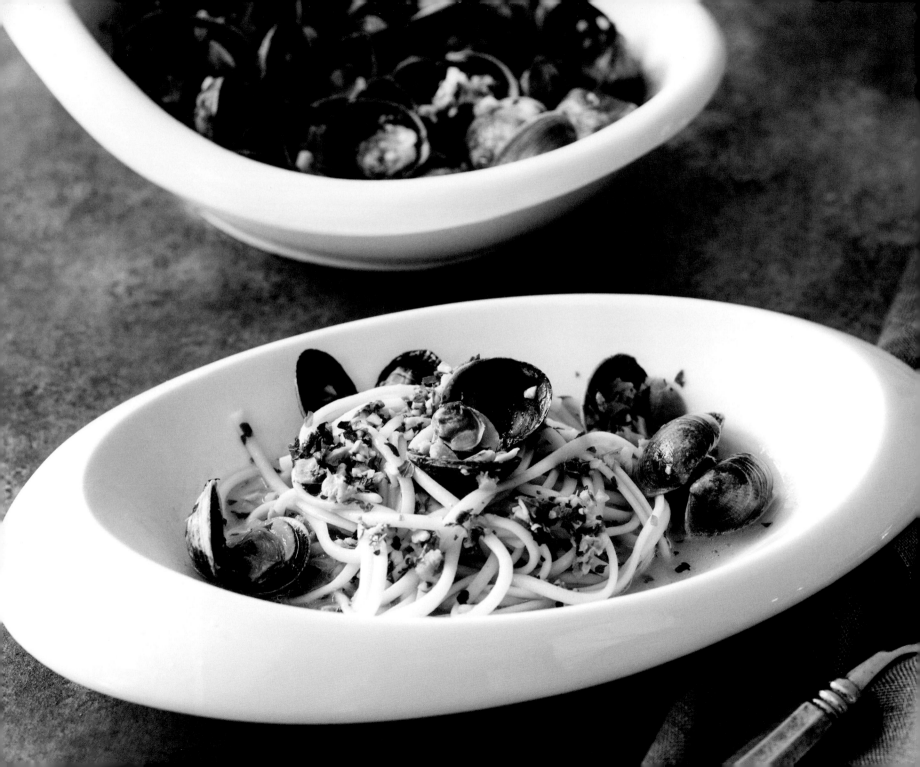

CHAPTER 6

Pasta

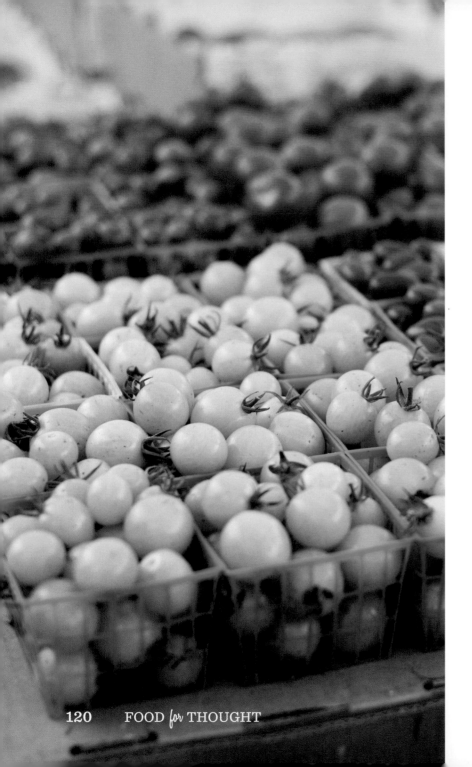

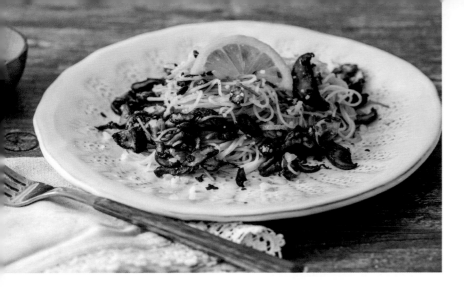

Angel Hair Pasta with Caramelized Mushrooms

SERVES 6 TO 8

INGREDIENTS

8 shiitaki mushrooms, stems removed and discarded, thinly sliced

1 (8-ounce) package white button or cremini mushrooms, a sliver of the bottom of each stem removed and discarded, thinly sliced

2 large portobello mushrooms, stems removed and discarded, chopped into 1-inch pieces

⅓ cup fresh lemon juice

⅓ cup extra-virgin olive oil

2 tablespoons shallots, peeled and finely chopped

5 garlic cloves, peeled and finely chopped

¼ teaspoon crushed red pepper

1 teaspoon each kosher salt and cracked black pepper

½ cup dry white wine

8 ounces angel hair pasta (see Cook's Note)

3 tablespoons finely chopped Italian (flat leaf) parsley

3 tablespoons lemon zest

½ cup freshly grated Parmesan cheese, plus 1 cup Romano cheese, combined

Crushed red pepper

INSTRUCTIONS

1. In a glass bowl toss the shiitake, white button, and portobello mushrooms and the the lemon juice.

2. Heat a large skillet on medium-high heat for 2 minutes. Add the olive oil, shallots, garlic, and crushed red pepper; sauté 1 minute. Add the marinated mushrooms, salt, and pepper; mix well.

3. The mushrooms will start to release a lot of liquid as they cook. Once that liquid has evaporated, about 6 to 8 minutes, they will start to caramelize and sizzle. When that occurs, add the white wine and cook down 6 minutes. Turn off the heat while you prepare the pasta.

4. Cook the pasta according to package directions. Drain.

5. Add the pasta to the mushroom mixture and increase the heat to medium-high. Use tongs to gently mix.

6. For each serving garnish with a sprinkling of the parsley, lemon zest, 2 to 3 tablespoons of the combined cheeses, and crushed red pepper.

Cook's Note: I prefer angel hair pasta with this sauce, but you can use any pasta you like. I have used farfalle, linguine, penne, and gluten-free pasta, all with good results.

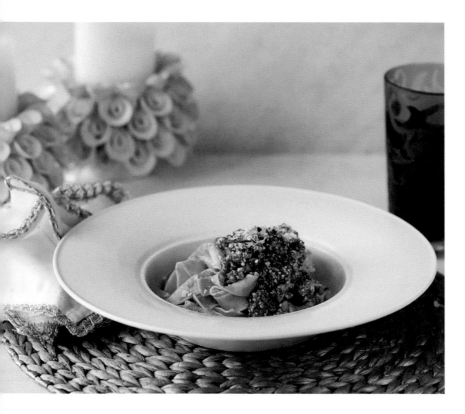

Heart-Healthy Pappardelle with Turkey Bolognese

SERVES 6 TO 8

INGREDIENTS

1 large white onion, peeled and quartered

1 small carrot, peeled and cut into four pieces

1 celery rib, cut into four pieces

⅓ cup extra-virgin olive oil

1½ pounds ground dark meat turkey

2 turkey sausages, casings removed

2 teaspoons kosher salt

1 cup low-fat milk or cashew milk

⅓ cup dry white wine

2 tablespoons tomato paste

1 (28-ounce) can tomato purée

1½ cups water, plus additional as needed

1 pound pappardelle pasta

3 cups freshly grated Parmesan cheese

½ cup coarsely chopped fresh basil

INSTRUCTIONS

1. In a food processor, process the onion until it's in small pieces. Remove onion and pulse the carrot and celery until they are finely chopped.

2. Heat a medium-sized saucepan on medium-high until it's hot; add the olive oil and heat 30 seconds. Add the chopped onion. Reduce the heat to medium, and sauté 2 minutes. Add the carrot and celery; sauté another 2 minutes.

3. Add the turkey and turkey sausage, using a metal spatula to break up the meat. Sprinkle with the salt and pour in the milk, continuing to break up the meat.

4. Cook until the meat starts to sizzle, about 10 minutes. Add the wine and mix well. Continue to cook until you hear a sizzle again.

5. Reduce the heat to a simmering boil. Add the tomato paste; stir in completely and keep mixing for at least 30 seconds.

6. Add the tomato purée, and water. Mix well. Cover and simmer on medium-low heat for 1 hour, stirring often. If the sauce is getting too thick, add more water, ¼ cup at a time.

7. Cook the pasta according to the package directions. Drain well and return it to its cooking pot.

8. Turn the heat to high, add several ladlesful of the sauce, and heat until the pasta and sauce are warmed through.

9. Serve in preheated pasta bowls. Sprinkle plenty of Parmesan cheese on top, and garnish with the basil. Serve immediately.

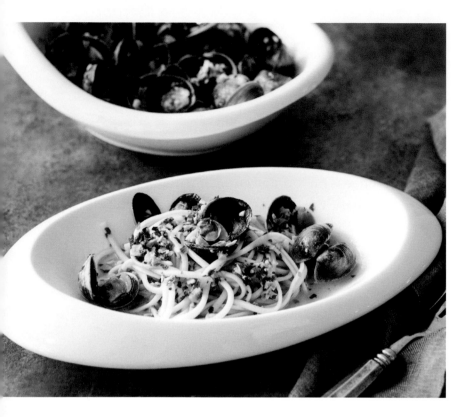

Linguine with Fresh Baby Manila Clams

Clams are mollusks that have a chewy texture and a briny ocean taste. They contain many vitamins and minerals and are considered lean protein because they are low in fat. Clams are also a good source of minerals, phosphorus, potassium, zinc, copper, manganese, and selenium, as well as being high in iron. We usually think of protein and calcium as the elements most important for health, but dietary minerals are essential for a variety of bodily functions, such as strong bones, teeth, blood, skin, hair, nerve function, and muscle development. Minerals are needed for the body to work properly.

Fresh clams should be alive when you purchase them and have a mild, ocean-fresh aroma. Watch for shells that are opened, which may indicate the clam is dead. However, if you tap the shells and they react by closing, then the clam is still alive.

SERVES 4 TO 6

INGREDIENTS

4 dozen fresh baby Manila clams

⅔ cup extra-virgin olive oil

6 garlic cloves, peeled and chopped into small pieces

¼ teaspoon crushed red pepper, plus extra for garnish

1 cup dry white wine

1 (8-ounce) bottle clam juice

2 (6½-ounce) cans minced clams in clam juice

¼ teaspoon kosher salt

8 ounces linguine

1 cup tightly packed Italian (flat leaf) parsley, finely chopped

1 lemon, cut into wedges

INSTRUCTIONS

1. Rinse the clams really well in cool water; drain in a colander.

2. Heat a medium-sized saucepan over medium-high heat for 30 seconds. Add the olive oil and heat for 1 minute. Add the garlic and crushed red pepper. Sauté until the garlic starts to turn slightly golden, which should happen almost immediately. Be careful and don't burn the garlic because it will make the sauce taste bitter. If this happens you need to discard it completely and start again.

3. Add white wine and clam juice and cook for 1 minute. Add the two cans of minced clams with the juice. Turn the heat to medium, and cook on a low boil for 10 minutes.

4. Add the Manila clams, cover with a lid, turn the heat slightly higher, and steam 5 to 8 minutes until all the clams are open. Remove and discard any clams that do not open.

5. Bring 4 quarts of water with 2 tablespoons of table salt to a boil in a large pasta pot. Add the linguine and cook the pasta al dente.

6. Drain the pasta well and put it back into the pot you boiled it in. Add the clam sauce and toss while heating through on medium heat for 1 minute.

7. Sprinkle the fresh parsley over the pasta and additional crushed red pepper.

8. Serve with a lemon wedge.

Tip: When the clams are cooked, their shells will open, indicating the clam is fine to eat. Any clams whose shells do not open after cooking should be discarded.

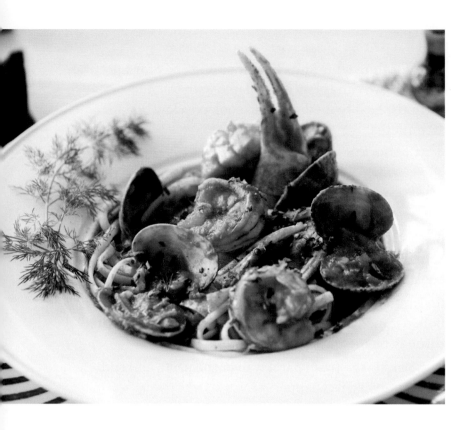

Linguine with Gifts from the Sea!

SERVES 6

INGREDIENTS

18 medium sized raw shrimp

18 Manila clams, rinsed and scrubbed well

18 small mussels (large ones are too tough), rinsed and scrubbed well, beards removed

6 crab claws, one for each serving

1 pound fresh cracked crab, cut into medium chunks

1 pound cod, sliced into 1-inch pieces

INSTRUCTIONS FOR THE GIFTS FROM THE SEA

1. Fill a large bowl with water and ice.

2. Use a paring knife to make a shallow slit along the back of the shrimps from head to tail. Pull out the black sand vein that runs along the center of the back. Rinse under cool water. Add to the bowl of ice water. Add the clams and mussels. Cover with plastic wrap and refrigerate until ready to use.

3. The seafood can be prepared 5 to 6 hours ahead providing you keep the fish in the refrigerator until you are ready to cook them.

SAUCE FOR THE LINGUINE

INGREDIENTS

⅓ cup extra-virgin olive oil

1 cup finely chopped white onions

6 scallions, white and light green parts, finely chopped

3 garlic cloves, peeled and thinly sliced

1 cup dry white wine

2 (28-ounce) cans crushed tomatoes in purée

1½ teaspoons kosher salt

½ teaspoon crushed red pepper

8 ounces linguine

¼ cup packed Italian (flat leaf) parsley, finely chopped

INSTRUCTIONS FOR THE LINGUINE

1. You can make the sauce up to two days before.

2. In a stockpot over medium-high heat add the olive oil. Heat for 30 seconds.

3. Reduce the heat to medium. Add the onions and scallions; sauté 8 minutes. Add the garlic; sauté 2 minutes. Pour in the wine and reduce the liquid by half. Add the tomatoes, salt, and crushed red pepper. Reduce the heat to low, simmering 45 minutes.

4. Increase the heat to medium-high. Add the mussels, clams, shrimps, crab claws, crab, and cod. Cook for 10 minutes or until all the clams and mussels have opened. Discard any mussels or clams that have not opened. Reduce the heat to a simmer while you prepare the pasta.

5. Cook the pasta according to the package directions. Drain the pasta, shaking it well drain any water. Transfer the pasta to the stockpot with the fish and seafood; mix well. Heat on high for 1 minute and serve!

6. Garnish with lots of fresh parsley!

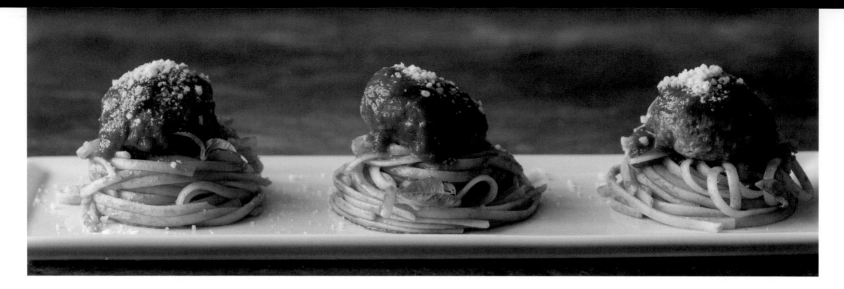

Pasta with Turkey Meatballs

I find using only turkey sausage for meatballs means they come out lighter and tastier than beef meatballs. You don't have to add lots of seasonings to the mix because the meatballs get their flavor from the seasoned sausage meat.

Prepare the sauce first, and while the sauce is simmering you can make the meatballs. After roasting the meatballs in the oven, they will finish cooking in the sauce. Doing it this way will keep the meatballs light and moist. Serve with your favorite pasta.

TURKEY MEATBALLS

MAKES 12 MEATBALLS

INGREDIENTS

6 (3-ounce) turkey sausages, casings removed

½ small white onion, peeled and cut into pieces

1 celery rib, cut into pieces

1 small carrot, peeled and cut into chunks

¼ cup loosely packed fresh Italian (flat leaf) parsley, coarsely chopped

1 cup regular or gluten-free Panko breadcrumbs

¼ cup freshly grated Parmesan cheese

¼ cup freshly grated Romano cheese

½ cup low fat milk or cashew milk

1 small garlic clove, crushed through a garlic press or finely minced

¼ teaspoon kosher salt

1 egg, lightly beaten

¼ cup ketchup

INSTRUCTIONS

1. Preheat the oven to 400F°.

2. Place the sausages in a medium-sized bowl. In a food processor, add the onion, celery, carrots, and parsley. Pulse-chop for 10 seconds. Using a spatula, push the mixture down the sides of the bowl and process 3 more seconds. Add the vegetable mixture to the sausage.

3. Add the breadcrumbs, Parmesan and Romano cheeses, milk, garlic, salt, egg, and ketchup. Use your hands to mix everything together until all the ingredients are combined.

4. Form 12 4-ounce meatballs using a ¼ dry measuring cup to help gauge the size of the meatball. Gently roll each one in your hands to make smooth, round balls. *Do not* pack them too tightly or they will be dry and not light once they're cooked. Place them on a baking sheet 3 inches apart. Bake 8 minutes; turn the meatballs over and bake another 4 minutes. *Do not* cook them all the way through; they will finish cooking in the sauce.

5. Bring the sauce up to a bubbling simmer. Carefully add the meatballs to the sauce and simmer on low for 30 minutes.

SAUCE FOR THE PASTA

SERVES 6

INGREDIENTS

⅓ cup extra-virgin olive oil

2 garlic cloves, peeled and smashed

1 (28-ounce) can tomato purée

½ teaspoon kosher salt

½ cup water

⅛ teaspoon crushed red pepper, plus additional for sprinkling

8 ounces of your favorite semolina or gluten-free pasta

½ cup freshly grated Romano cheese

INSTRUCTIONS

1. Heat a saucepan on medium-high heat for 30 seconds. Add the olive oil and garlic; sauté until the garlic starts to turn lightly golden, about 2 to 3 minutes. Be careful not to burn the garlic or the sauce will taste bitter; if this happens, discard the garlic and start again.

2. Add the tomato purée, salt, water, and crushed red pepper.

3. Lower the heat and simmer for 30 minutes. If the sauce is getting too thick, add water, ¼ cup at a time.

4. Once it is done simmering, you want it to have a silky consistency. Turn off heat and set aside while you make the meatballs.

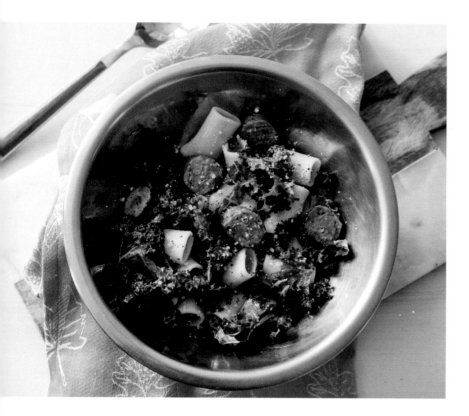

Pasta with Kale, White Beans, and Sausage

This recipe for kale pasta salad is one of my favorites and my family loves it! It's a great dish to take on a picnic, for a buffet, or to serve for Sunday brunch.

I am an outspoken advocate of "gut health" and I believe very strongly in consuming anti-inflammatory foods and drinks. That is why I include a lot of kale in my diet. I use it in smoothies, soups, sandwiches, and salads.

Here are some findings about the most beneficial properties of eating kale and why it is such a powerful anti-inflammatory agent. Most Western diets have an excess of Omega-6 fatty acids and a lack of Omega-3 fatty acids, which does not reflect the diet with which humans evolved. Omega-6s are inflammatory, and widespread consumption has been linked to many inflammation-related diseases, including rheumatoid arthritis, Chron's, and even some cancers. The introduction of kale to a more mainstream diet has helped to promote balance between Omega-6s and -3s, because kale has nearly a 1:1 ratio. It has slightly more Omega-3s, which can help to offset the negative effects of a diet rich in Omega-6s.

SERVES 6 TO 8

INGREDIENTS

5 organic hot or mild turkey sausages

8 ounces farfalle (bowtie) pasta

1 tablespoon extra-virgin olive oil

1 bunch kale, leaves torn off the stems and stems discarded

1 medium ripe avocado, peeled, pitted, and cut into chunks

Shallot Vinaigrette (see recipe, p. 208)

1 (15-ounce) can white navy beans, drained and
   rinsed throughly

½ teaspoon each kosher salt and cracked black pepper

3 tablespoons fresh lemon juice

1 cup freshly grated Parmesan cheese

¼ cup pomegranate seeds

2 tablespoons lemon zest

2 lemons, sliced into wedges

INSTRUCTIONS

1. Preheat the oven to 450F°.

2. On a rimmed baking sheet, roast the sausages for 30 minutes, turning them over after 15 minutes. Remove the sausages from the oven and cover lightly with foil. Set aside until you're ready to use them.

3. Cook the pasta according to package directions. Rinse with cool water and drain well, shaking the colander to eliminate all excess water. Transfer to a pasta bowl, drizzle the olive oil over the top, and mix.

4. In a separate salad bowl add the kale and avocado. Using your hands massage the avocado onto the kale leaves until they're coated completely.

5. Add the pasta into the bowl with the kale, 5 tablespoons of the Shallot Vinaigrette, beans, salt, pepper, and lemon juice; toss gently. Season by adding more salt and pepper if necessary.

6. Slice the sausages into 2 inch pieces. Scatter the sausages around the bowl. Sprinkle the Parmesan cheese, pomegranate seeds, and lemon zest over the top.

7. Serve with a lemon wedge.

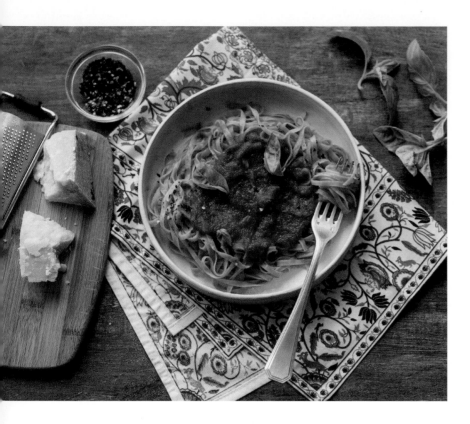

Fresh Roma Tomato Sauce

This is my all-time favorite tomato sauce. Anytime you can make a sauce using fresh tomatoes, I highly recommend it. Fresh tomatoes make a sauce sweeter and taste just like you would experience if you ordered pasta in Italy—authentic!

Tomatoes are a powerful antioxidant and contain vitamins A and C. These vitamins act as an antioxidant, working to neutralize dangerous free radicals in the bloodstream that can damage cells. The redder the tomato, the more beta-carotene and heart-healthy lycopene it contains. Look for tomatoes that are vibrantly colored with firm, shiny skins. Never refrigerate tomatoes; doing so will kill the flavor for sure, so keep them at room temperature.

You can also use this sauce as a soup. Just add 2 cups vegetable or chicken stock to thin it. Serve hot or chilled!

SERVES 4 TO 6

INGREDIENTS

⅓ cup extra-virgin olive oil

1 medium yellow onion, peeled and chopped into medium chunks

6 scallions, white and green parts, chopped into small chunks

½ cup white wine

16 ripe medium-sized Roma tomatoes, quartered

2 teaspoons each kosher salt and cracked black pepper

¼ teaspoon crushed red pepper, plus more for garnish

8 ounces of your favorite pasta

1 cup freshly grated Parmesan cheese

8 basil leaves

INSTRUCTIONS

1. Heat a large heavy saucepan on medium-high heat for 2 minutes.

2. Add the olive oil and swirl to cover the bottom of the pan. Immediately add the onions and scallions; cook 8 minutes to bring out the juices and natural sugars in the onions.

3. Add the wine; cook until the liquid is reduced by half. Add the tomatoes, salt, pepper, and crushed red pepper if desired. Mix well, then lower the heat to medium.

4. Cover the saucepan, making sure the lid is slightly ajar. Simmer on medium heat for 50 minutes to cook down the liquid from the tomatoes, until the sauce has thickened. Check every 10 minutes or so to make sure the tomatoes are still at a simmer and not boiling.

5. Place half of the tomato mixture into a blender and process for 1 minute.

6. Pass the mixture through a chinois (strainer) into a clean pot to remove the tomato skins and seeds. Repeat this process until all of the tomatoes have been blended and strained. Season, adding more salt and pepper, if desired.

7. Cook your favorite pasta according to package directions. While the pasta is boiling turn the sauce to medium heat. When the pasta is ready, drain it really well. Pour the drained pasta back into the pot in which it was cooked.

8. Increase the heat to high and add three ladlesful of the sauce. Mix to evenly distribute the sauce with the pasta and to heat through.

9. Add a serving of the pasta into each preheated bowl. Ladle more sauce over the top. Garnish with the Parmesan cheese, basil, and a pinch of crushed red pepper.

Cook's Note: Remember to warm your pasta bowls with hot water just before serving to take the chill off. If you don't have a chinois to strain the tomatoes, use a strainer with holes large enough to catch the tomato seeds and skins. If the holes are too tightly meshed the sauce will be thin and watery.

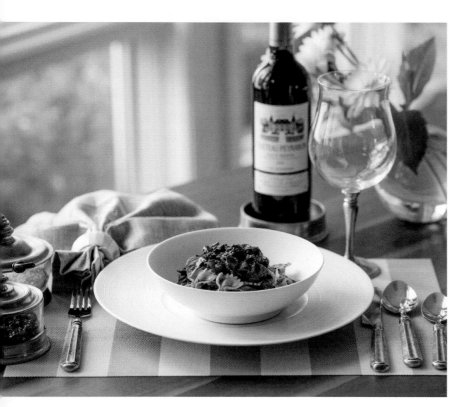

Meatless "Meat" Sauce!

Even if you aren't a vegetarian you will love this sauce. It's full of meaty flavor without using any meat. It's made with three different kinds of immune-fighting mushrooms, each with their own flavor and specific antioxidants. If you add a pinch of fennel seeds to the sauce it will taste like a meat sauce made with sausages. Try it—you won't be disappointed!

SERVES 6 TO 8

INGREDIENTS

½ cup extra-virgin olive oil

½ yellow onion, peeled and finely diced

3 shallots, peeled and finely diced

4 garlic cloves, peeled and finely diced

2 large (4 ounces each) Portobello mushrooms, stems removed and discarded, finely chopped

12 shiitake mushrooms, stems removed and discarded, finely chopped

2 (8-ounce) packages white or brown button mushrooms, stems removed and discarded, finely chopped

1 teaspoon each kosher salt and cracked black pepper

½ cup red wine

1 (6-ounce) can tomato paste

1 teaspoon fennel seed, optional

2 cups water

8 ounces of your favorite pasta

1 cup freshly grated Romano cheese

1 cup freshly grated Parmesan cheese

¼ cup finely chopped Italian (flat leaf) parsley

Crushed red pepper

INSTRUCTIONS

1. Heat a large cast-iron or heavy bottom skillet on medium-high heat for 1 minute. Add the olive oil, onion, and shallots. Lower the heat to medium, and sauté, stirring frequently, 5 minutes. Add the garlic; sauté 2 minutes more.

2. Add the Portobello mushrooms and sauté 5 minutes. Add the shiitake mushrooms and sauté 3 minutes. Add the button mushrooms, salt, and pepper; stir.

3. After 5 minutes the mushrooms will start to release their liquids. Cook until the liquid has almost evaporated and you hear a sizzle. Keep turning the mushrooms over to caramelize them until they have turned a deep rich brown.

4. Pour in the wine and cook it down for 5 minutes. Add the tomato paste and the fennel seeds (if you're using them). Reduce the heat to medium-low and cook 3 minutes, stirring often. Add the 2 cups of water and stir; turn the heat to low and simmer 30 minutes.

5. Cook the pasta according to package directions. Before you drain the pasta, save 1 cup of the pasta water.

6. Drain the pasta and add it to the skillet with the mushrooms. Increase the heat to high. Mix everything thoroughly and heat through. Add the reserved pasta water, Parmesan and Romano cheese, and the parsley. Mix well. Garnish with the crushed red pepper and more Parmesan and Romano cheese! Serve immediately.

Cook's Note: To clean mushrooms, use a damp paper towel or a mushroom brush to wipe each mushroom, one at time, to remove the dirt. Don't soak mushrooms in water. If you rinse them in water, make sure to dry them well with a paper towel. Mushrooms won't brown and caramelize nicely if they are damp.

Tomato Sauce in the Raw

6 TO 8 SERVINGS

INGREDIENTS

3 pounds baby organic red and yellow Roma tomatoes,
   sliced lengthwise

⅓ cup extra-virgin olive oil

½ cup freshly grated Parmesan cheese,
   plus more for serving

½ cup freshly grated Romano cheese,
   plus more for serving

1 cup coarsely chopped Italian (flat leaf) parsley

2 garlic cloves, smashed

12 fresh basil leaves, stacked on top of one another,
   rolled tightly and then sliced into thin ribbons

8 ounces penne or farfalle (butterfly-shaped) pasta

1 teaspoon each kosher salt and cracked black pepper

¼ cup Kalamata olives, for garnish

½ teaspoon crushed red pepper flakes, for garnish

INSTRUCTIONS

1. Place the tomatoes, olive oil, Parmesan cheese, Romano cheese, parsley, garlic, and basil into a large pasta bowl. Toss to mix well.

2. Cover tightly with plastic wrap and let it sit at room temperature 1 to 2 hours. The longer the tomatoes sit at room temperature, the better, as this will give some time for all the flavors to marry.

3. Cook the pasta according to the package directions *and don't forget to salt the water*. When the pasta is *al dente* drain and rinse gently in cool water. Shake vigorously to drain all of the water.

4. Find and remove the garlic cloves from the tomatoes, saving them for another use. Transfer the pasta into the bowl with the tomatoes, add salt and pepper, and toss to mix well.

5. Garnish with Kalamata olives and crushed red pepper flakes.

6. Sprinkle more Parmesan and Romano cheeses on top!

Cook's Note: *Al dente* refers to the degree of doneness of properly cooked pasta. The term *al dente* comes from an Italian phrase which translates as "to the tooth." When cooked *al dente*, pasta should be tender but still firm to the bite.

Tip: If you can't find baby Roma tomatoes, use cherry tomatoes.

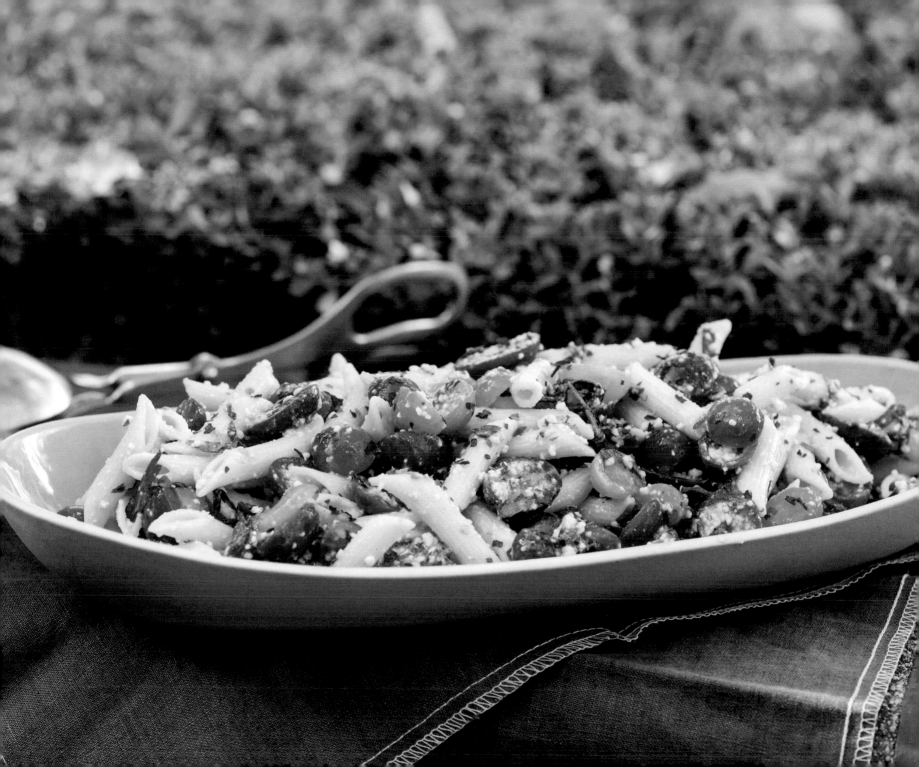

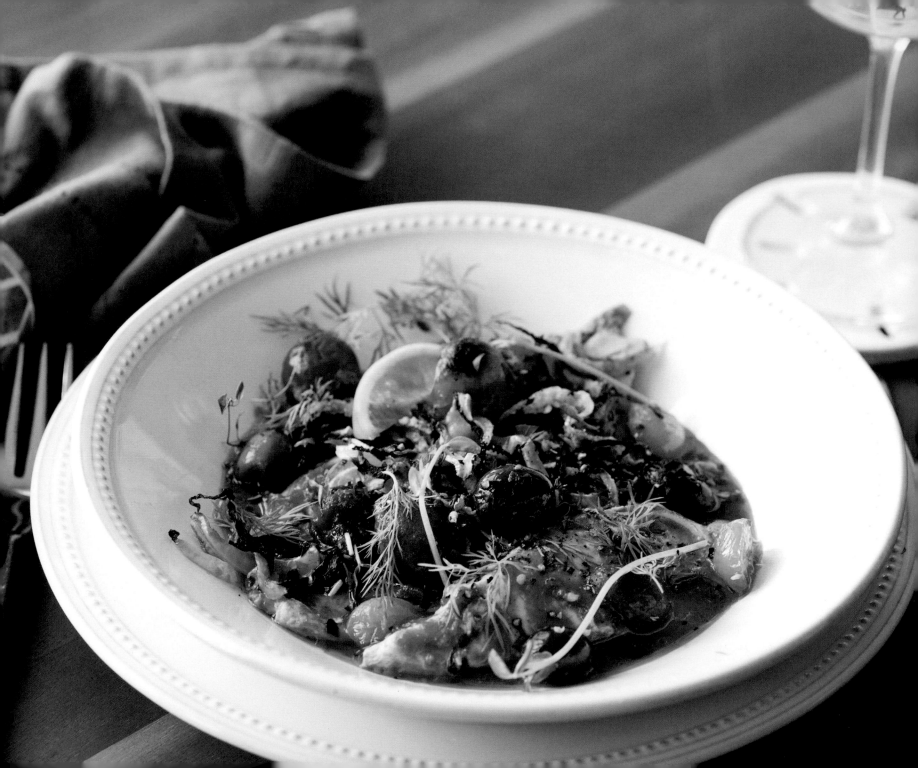

CHAPTER 7

Gifts from the Sea

I have always loved fish, even as a child. Being raised as Catholic Italians, we of course, had fish every Friday night. When my Nonna was living with us, it was a feast to behold every time we sat down on Fridays to have dinner. She served dishes originating from the coastal village where she grew up, and the fish she served was always purchased fresh from our fishmonger, even in the winter, in Cleveland where I grew up. Our home had the aromas of garlic bathing in olive oil, simmering fresh tomatoes, and fish cooking without that fishy smell. Go figure. So it should not be a surprise that I have continued to prepare, serve, and enjoy fish at least twice a week.

The American Heart Association recommends eating fish at least two times (two servings) a week. Each serving is 3.5 ounce cooked, or about ¾ cup of flaked fish. Fish is filled with omega-3 fatty acids. Omega-3 fatty acid is a class of essential fatty acids found in fish oil, especially salmon, halibut, and other cold water fish. They help lower cholesterol levels in the blood. You have to get them through the foods you eat since the body can't make them on its own.

Try to avoid fish that contain high levels of mercury, such as mackerel, marlin, orange roughy, shark, swordfish, ahi tuna, and big eye tuna.

I've also included recipes for shellfish, such as mussels, clams, shrimp, and crab. These have an impressive nutritional profile and give you a shot of important minerals, like zinc, which help build immunity. I thought very carefully about what recipes I created for this chapter on "gifts from the sea." Each dish is a labor of love that I carry in my heart from the beautiful memories I have watching my Nonna prepare those Friday night meals.

Broiled Miso-Glazed Sea Bass in Lemongrass Coconut Thai Broth

This is my very favorite recipe for fish—ever. It's light, delicate, and full of flavor. The buttery sea bass is infused with Asian flavors and nearly melts in your mouth. The broth is a balance of sweet coconut and citrus, with a hint of heat that is pleasing to your senses of smell and taste. It's delicious on its own, but sometimes I will add lime-infused brown rice and a vegetable—my choice is sautéed bok choy.

I've included the recipes for the Miso Glaze, Coconut Thai Broth, and the Chile Garnish. You'll need to make the glaze and broth first for this recipe.

MISO GLAZE

SERVES 4

INGREDIENTS

4 (6-ounce) sea bass fillets

3 tablespoons light soy sauce

3 tablespoons dry white wine

1 tablespoon honey

2 tablespoons yellow miso paste

INSTRUCTIONS FOR THE GLAZE

1. Whisk the soy sauce, wine, honey, and miso paste.

2. Pour the marinade over the sea bass fillets and turn them to coat all sides. Cover the baking dish tightly with plastic wrap; refrigerate to chill. After one hour flip the fillets over and chill for another hour. The fillets can be left it in the marinade for up to 5 hours.

COCONUT THAI BROTH

INGREDIENTS

3 tablespoons extra-virgin olive oil

3 scallions, white and light green parts, chopped in thirds

2 garlic cloves, peeled and smashed

3 pieces ginger, each 1-inch thick, chopped

1 serrano chili, sliced in quarters from top of chili to bottom, so you end up with 4 strips

2 tablespoons fresh lime juice, reserve the rind

1 stalk lemongrass, woody part removed, sliced open lengthwise, then cut in half, and rinsed

1½ quarts water

2 teaspoons kosher salt

1 (15-ounce) can coconut cream

Recipe continues ▶

1. Heat a medium-sized stockpot on medium-high heat for 2 minutes.

2. Add the olive oil, scallions, garlic, ginger, and serrano chili; sauté 1 minute.

3. Add the lime juice, lime rind, lemongrass, water, salt, and Coconut Cream. Stir until there are no lumps from the coconut cream.

4. Bring to a boil; reduce the heat to low and simmer for 1 hour.

5. Strain the broth and pour back into the stockpot. If you're not serving right away, pour into a glass container or jar, cover tightly with a lid, and refrigerate until ready to use; it will keep for up to 2 days.

CHILE GARNISH

INGREDIENTS

1 serrano chili, quartered
⅓ cup finely chopped cilantro or Italian (flat leaf) parsley
3 scallions, white and light green parts, chopped small
2 tablespoons toasted sesame seeds

INSTRUCTIONS

Combine the above ingredients and sprinkle on top of the sea bass before serving. Divide equally among servings.

BROILED SEA BASS

INSTRUCTIONS

1. Remove the marinated sea bass fillets from the refrigerator. Let them sit on the counter at room temperature for 30 minutes.

2. This is a good time to prepare the garnish. Mix together the serrano chili, cilantro or parsley, scallions, and sesame seeds. Set aside.

3. After 30 minutes, pre-heat the broiler on high.

4. Pour the olive oil onto a baking sheet and use a paper towel to coat the pan. Lay the fillets on the baking sheet 3 inches apart.

5. Broil 4 inches from the heat source for 10 minutes until they're caramelized. Do not turn them over.

6. Keep your eyes on the fillets and check every minute to make sure they're not burning. Remove from broiler and let them rest 5 minutes.

TO ASSEMBLE

1. Bring the broth to a boil, lower heat to a simmer.

2. While broth is heating, rinse the serving bowls in hot water to take the chill off; this will keep the broth hot.

3. Add a ladle of hot broth in the pre-heated soup bowls. Lay in the sea bass.

4. At this point you can add rice or vegetables to the bowl, if you are including them.

5. Add garnish, dividing equally among servings.

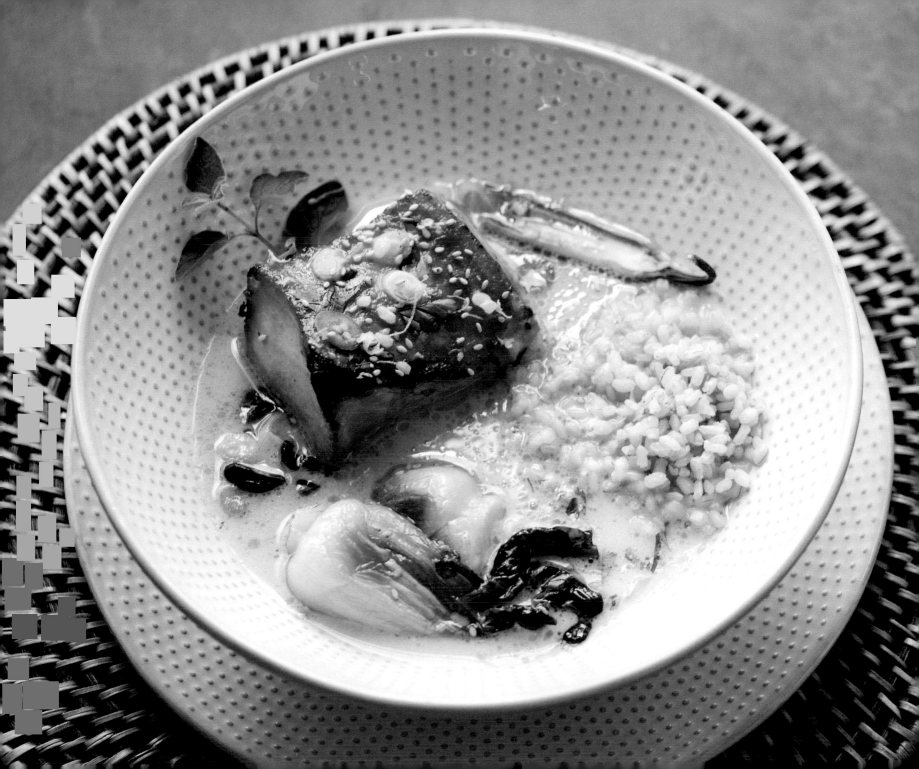

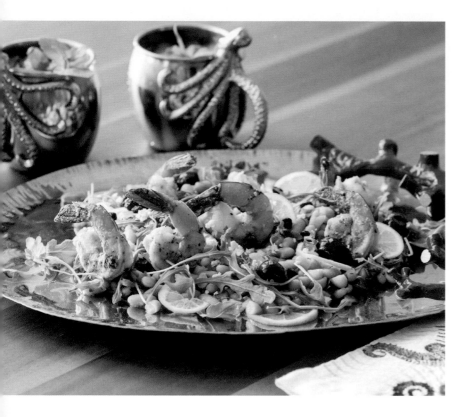

Roasted Shrimp with Navy Beans and Garden Greens

This is a perfect dish for a light lunch or dinner as a first course served with tomato soup, hot or chilled.

SERVES 4

INGREDIENTS

12 large shrimp, peeled and deveined (see Cook's Note)

¼ cup, plus 3 tablespoons extra-virgin olive oil, divided

1½ teaspoon each kosher salt and cracked black pepper, divided

1 teaspoon garlic powder

1 teaspoon onion powder

6 fresh sage leaves, torn into pieces

2 (15-ounce) cans Navy beans, rinsed gently and drained

⅓ cup fresh lemon juice

¼ cup Italian (flat leaf) parsley, coarsely chopped

6 fresh basil leaves, rolled tightly and thinly sliced

5 mint leaves, chopped

2 cups baby arugula

2 cups baby spinach, chopped

2 cups frisée lettuce, torn into small pieces

12 Kalamata olives

1 cup Greek or French feta cheese, crumbled

1 lemon, thinly sliced

4 tablespoons pomegranate seeds (in season)

INSTRUCTIONS

1. Preheat the oven to 375F°.

2. In a glass bowl add the shrimp, 3 tablespoons olive oil, 1 teaspoon salt, 1 teaspoon pepper, garlic powder, and onion powder. Mix well and let stand 15 minutes.

3. On a baking sheet arrange the shrimp in one layer, 2 inches apart. Spread the sage leave pieces over the top; roast 12 minutes. Remove from the oven and cover lightly with foil.

FOR THE SALAD

1. Combine in a glass bowl the navy beans, ½ teaspoon salt, ½ teaspoon pepper, ¼ cup olive oil, lemon juice, parsley, basil, mint, arugula, and frisée lettuce. Mix gently.

2. Arrange the bean salad on a large platter and top with the roasted shrimp. Add the Kalamata olives, feta, lemon slices, and pomegranate seeds.

Cook's Note: To peel and devein raw shrimp, start underneath where the legs are attached. Hold the shrimp firmly by its tail and pull off the shell, leaving the tail intact. Make a shallow slit down the middle of the back; you will see the black intestine. Under running water remove the intestine by lifting out the black vein. Use your hands to pull it out. Turn the shrimp over and do the same with the underbelly, removing the white vein.

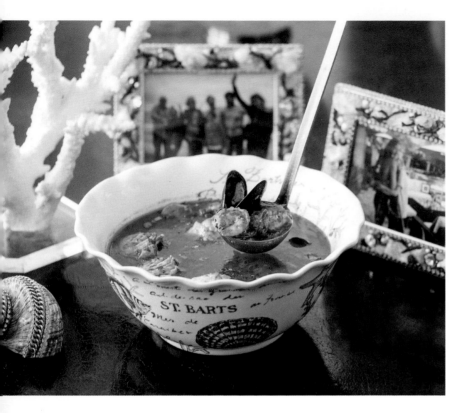

Heavenly Saffron Broth with Gifts from the Sea

SERVES 6

INGREDIENTS

1 pound cod, sliced into 3-inch pieces

1 dozen medium-sized raw shrimp, shelled and deveined

1 dozen mussels, rinsed, scrubbed, and beards removed (see Cook's Note)

2 dozen baby Manila clams, rinsed well

¼ cup extra-virgin olive oil

4 cloves garlic, minced

½ cup dry white wine

1 (8-ounce) bottle clam juice

1 (28-ounce) can diced tomatoes in purée

2 cups vegetable broth

1½ teaspoons kosher salt

¼ teaspoon cayenne pepper

1 tablespoon saffron threads

1 dozen medium scallops, side tendons removed

1 cup packed Italian (flat leaf) parsley, finely chopped

2 tablespoons lemon zest

1 sourdough baguette

Spicy Mayo (see recipe, opposite)

INSTRUCTIONS

1. In a large bowl, add the shrimp, mussels, and clams. Fill the bowl with cold water and 2 cups ice. Cover and refrigerate until you're ready to cook.

2. In a large stockpot over medium-high heat, add the olive oil; heat 1 minute. Add the garlic and sauté 2 minutes or until the garlic starts to turn golden. Add the wine; cook 30 seconds. Add the clam juice and tomatoes. Reduce the heat to medium-low and simmer gently for 30 minutes.

3. Add the vegetable broth, salt, cayenne pepper, and saffron threads. Simmer 30 more minutes, stirring occasionally, until the sauce starts to thicken.

4. Bring the sauce up to a low boil, on medium high heat. Add mussels and clams. Cover with a lid and cook 2 minutes.

5. Add the cod, shrimp, and scallops; cook 6 minutes. Discard any mussels or clams that remain closed.

TO ASSEMBLE

Ladle soup into an individual deep bowl along with a generous dollop of the spicy mayo. Garnish with parsley and lemon zest, to taste. Serve with sourdough bread on the side and dip it into the broth!

Cook's Note: Before you cook raw mussels, check to make sure none have opened. If any have opened, tap the shell; if it closes and remains closed, you can use the mussel. If it stays open, the mussel is dead. Discard it.

Tip: Keep the cod pieces covered and refrigerated until needed.

Suggestion: Fish stew or bouillabaisse is traditionally served with *rouille*. It adds intense flavor and texture to the dish. The rouille can be made a day ahead and stored in the refrigerator overnight until ready to serve. If you choose to make a rouille, there are many recipes available online.

SPICY MAYO

INGREDIENTS

1 (12-ounce) jar roasted red peppers
2 garlic cloves, peeled
½ teaspoon paprika
1 tablespoon fresh lemon juice
1 cup low-fat mayonnaise
¼ teaspoon kosher salt
¼ teaspoon cayenne pepper

INSTRUCTIONS

In a blender or food processor, place the red peppers, garlic, paprika, lemon juice, mayonnaise, salt, and cayenne pepper. Blend until smooth. Cover.

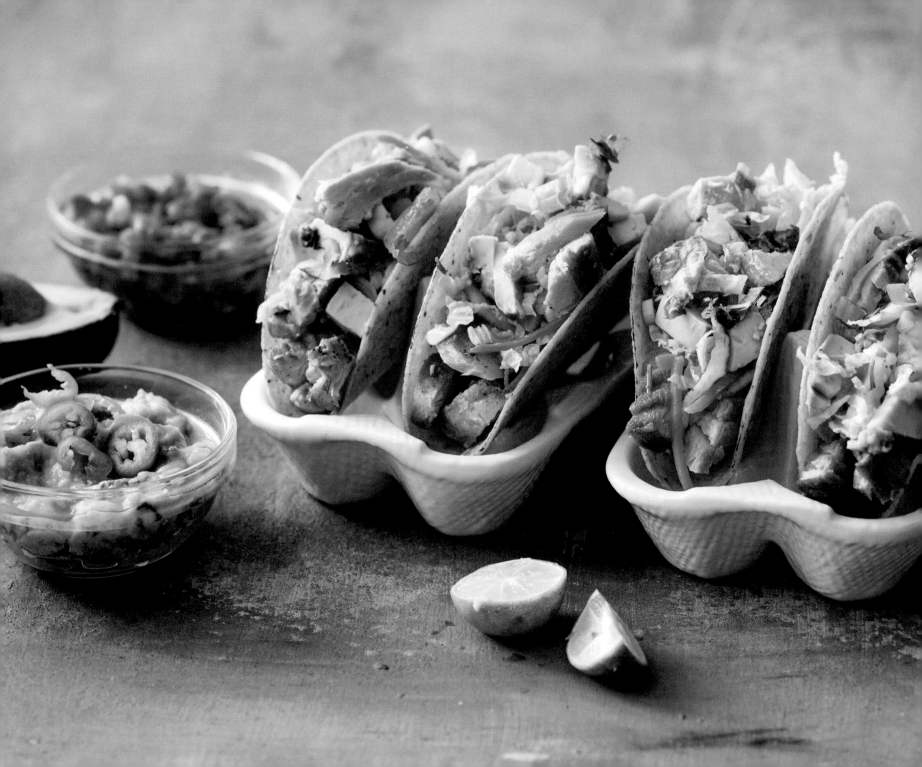

Grilled Salmon Tacos with Cilantro-Lime Slaw

There are a few steps needed to make these tacos, but I feel that these are worth the extra effort. I love to make tacos out of just about everything! Salmon is my all-time favorite fish to eat, not to mention how good it is for you.

Most of the steps for this recipe can be done the day before. I've organized everything to make it easy and simple, starting with the ingredients you will need. Don't let this long list scare you; most of them are pantry items that you probably already have. So double-check before you shop. Make your own list of ingredients to buy according to what you already have in stock.

You can use either the hard shell or soft tortillas to make this dish.

CILANTRO-LIME SLAW

INGREDIENTS

1 (1-pound) bag organic slaw mix (shredded cabbage and carrot)

2 tablespoons mayonnaise

3 tablespoons extra-virgin olive oil

¼ cup fresh lime juice

1 tablespoon apple cider vinegar

2 tablespoons seasoned rice vinegar

1 teaspoon kosher salt

2 tablespoons finely chopped cilantro

3 scallions, chopped small

INSTRUCTIONS

1. Make sure to rinse the bagged slaw mix even though the bag may say it's already rinsed. Spin dry or roll in paper towel to dry.

2. Place the slaw in a bowl.

3. In a separate bowl whisk the mayonnaise, olive oil, lime juice, apple cider vinegar, rice vinegar, salt, cilantro, and scallions. Pour the dressing over the slaw and toss well. Cover and place in the refrigerator until ready to use.

Recipe continues ▶

TOMATO SALSA

INGREDIENTS

12 Roma tomatoes
½ cup red onion, chopped small
¼ cup cilantro chopped small
2 scallions, finely chopped
2 tablespoons fresh lime juice
1 teaspoon kosher salt
1 jalapeño finely diced with the seeds
2 tablespoons extra-virgin olive oil

INSTRUCTIONS

1. Slice each tomato lengthwise; remove seeds and core. Then, slice the tomato into strips and cut into ¼-inch pieces.

2. Place the tomatoes, red onion, cilantro, scallions, lime juice, salt, jalapeño, and olive oil in a glass bowl, and mix well.

3. Cover in an airtight glass container and place in the refrigerator for at least 3 to 4 hours.

4. Salsa can be made the day before and will last 3 days in the refrigerator in an airtight container.

SRIRACHA MAYO

INGREDIENTS

⅓ cup Sriracha hot sauce
½ cup regular or vegan mayonnaise

INSTRUCTIONS

In a small bowl combine the Sriracha and mayonnaise; mix well. Pour into a needle nose bottle and refrigerate until ready to use.

GUACAMOLE

INGREDIENTS

4 ripe avocados peeled, pitted (reserve 1 pit)
3 tablespoons fresh lime juice
¼ cup white onion diced small
1 jalapeño, seeds included, diced small
¼ cup finely chopped cilantro
1 teaspoon kosher salt
¼ cup lemon juice

INSTRUCTIONS

1. In a glass mixing bowl, add the avocados and use a potato masher to crush them into chunks. Add all of the rest of the ingredients and use a wooden spoon to mix together until combined.

2. If you don't serve the guacamole immediately, add the avocado pit in the middle of guacamole, cover tightly with plastic wrap and place in the refrigerator until ready to serve. Can be made up to 3 hours in advance and kept chilled.

GRILLED SALMON TACOS

INGREDIENTS

8 hard taco shells or soft tortillas

2 teaspoons ground cumin

1 teaspoon chili powder

1 teaspoon garlic powder

1 teaspoon onion powder

1 teaspoon kosher salt

1 lb. wild caught salmon

3 tablespoons extra-virgin olive oil

Cilantro Slaw (see recipe, p. 149)

Tomato Salsa (see recipe, opposite)

Sriracha Mayo (see recipe, opposite)

Guacamole (see recipe, opposite)

1 jalapeño, seeds included, diced small

¼ cup finely chopped cilantro

4 cups shredded Monterey Jack cheese

4 fresh limes, cut into wedges

INSTRUCTIONS

1. Preheat oven to 200°F.

2. Hang the taco shells over the grates of the oven rack to heat them. If using soft tortillas wrap in kitchen towel and place in the oven.

3. Whisk the cumin, chili powder, garlic, onion powder, and salt. Rub the spice mixture on top and sides of salmon, not the skin side.

4. Heat a cast iron skillet or heavy bottom skillet on medium-high heat for 3 minutes until hot. Add the olive oil and immediately place the salmon skin side down and cook without disturbing for 4 minutes.

5. Turn salmon over and cook for 3 more minutes.

6. Salmon will be medium pink in the center. If you wish to make it well done, turn heat to medium and cook 2 more minutes on each side.

7. Remove the fish and place it on a cutting board, tent with foil and allow it to rest for 10 minutes. Slice the salmon in chunks.

TO ASSEMBLE

1. Remove the Cilantro Slaw from the refrigerator and drain the excess liquid. Take out the Sriracha mayo and guacamole and place on the counter.

2. Remove the taco shells from the oven and prop them up in a taco holder. I used my ceramic egg holder to prop mine.

3. Take a warm taco shell, add several pieces of salmon on bottom of shell. Add 3 tablespoons guacamole over the salmon. Spread a serving of slaw, a sprinkle of cilantro and jalapeño, as much as you want, and a healthy squiggle of the Sriracha mayo over the top.

4. Serve with salsa and sliced lime wedges on the side!

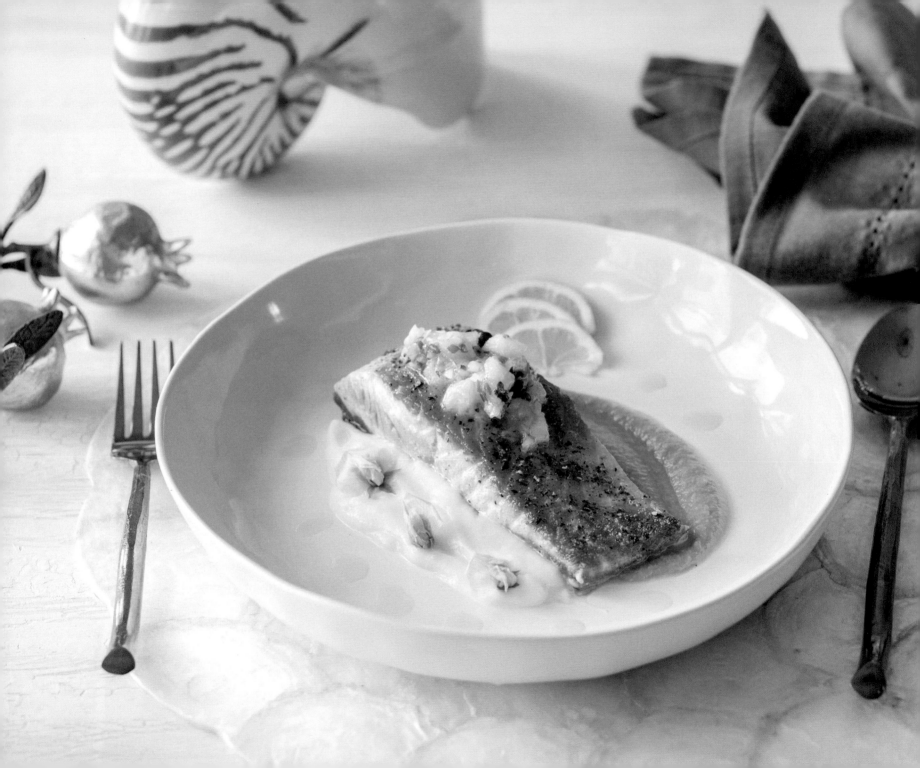

Roasted Crusted Salmon with Cauliflower and Pea Purée

My recipes are usually really easy to follow and quick to make without having to go through many steps to achieve success. Having said that, there are a few steps you have to go through to bring this dish together. I promise you it is so worth the effort. I will give you a few tips to make it easier. But please don't bypass this one.

This recipe for Roasted Salmon and the Broiled Miso-glazed Sea Bass are two of my most prized recipes and my favorite dishes ever! Here are a few suggestions to follow to make putting this together a breeze.

If you make the ghee, Spicy Mango Salsa, Cauliflower Purée (so easy), and Pea Purée (even easier) the day before, all you have to do when you serve this dish is reheat the cauliflower and pea purées, and prepare the salmon, which takes 10 to 15 minutes. Just look at the photo to see how beautiful this dish is. You will be so proud to serve it to your family and guests!

CAULIFLOWER PURÉE

INGREDIENTS

1 large head cauliflower, cut up
2 garlic cloves, peeled and smashed
1 tablespoon extra-virgin olive oil
1 tablespoon kosher salt
2 tablespoons caper juice, from a jar of capers

INSTRUCTIONS

1. In a stockpot over high heat add the cauliflower. Cover with water; add the garlic, olive oil, and kosher salt. Bring the water to a boil and boil the cauliflower 15 minutes or until it's soft and tender. Before you drain the cauliflower, reserve 1 cup of the cooking water and the garlic.

2. Drain the cauliflower. Place it in a blender, and add the reserved garlic, caper juice, and ½ cup of the reserved cauliflower cooking water. Blend for 30 seconds. If the cauliflower purée looks too thick, add more cauliflower water, ¼ cup at a time, to get a whipped, creamy consistency (like creamy mashed potatoes).

Recipe continues ▶

PEA PURÉE

INGREDIENTS

1 cup vegetable stock

1 (1-pound) bag organic frozen petite peas

½ teaspoon kosher salt

INSTRUCTIONS

In a medium-sized saucepan, bring the vegetable stock to a boil. Add the peas and salt; cook 2 minutes. Pour into a blender and process 30 seconds until it's smooth and creamy.

SPICY MANGO SALSA

INGREDIENTS

1 ripe mango (1 cup) peeled, pitted, and chopped into small pieces

1 cucumber, peeled, seeded, and diced

1 tablespoon finely diced jalapeño, seeds removed, optional

¼ cup red bell pepper, seeded and diced

¼ teaspoon crushed red pepper

1 scallion trimmed, cut into thin rings

2 tablespoons extra-virgin olive oil

2 tablespoons fresh lime juice

½ teaspoon kosher salt

2 teaspoons cilantro, finely chopped

6 mint leaves, finely chopped

INSTRUCTIONS

Place the mango, cucumber, jalapeño, bell pepper, crushed red pepper, scallion, olive oil, lime juice, salt, cilantro, and mint in a glass bowl or Mason jar. Mix thoroughly. Cover tightly and refrigerate. This salsa will last up to 3 days.

ROASTED SALMON

SERVES 4

INGREDIENTS

4 (5-ounce) wild salmon fillets

2 teaspoons each kosher salt and cracked black pepper

¼ cup Ghee (see recipe, p. 222)

2 tablespoons extra-virgin olive oil

Cauliflower Purée (see recipe, p. 153)

Pea Purée (see recipe, opposite)

Spicy Mango Salsa (see recipe, opposite)

2 tablespoons avocado oil

1 lemon, thinly sliced

Edible flowers (available online; optional)

INSTRUCTIONS

1. Preheat the oven to 450F°. Place the oven rack in the middle of the oven.

2. Sprinkle both sides of the salmon fillets with the salt and pepper.

3. Heat a cast-iron skillet for 2 minutes on high heat. Add the ghee and olive oil; swirl to coat the bottom of the skillet. Add the salmon, skin side down. Turn the heat to medium-high, cook for 4 minutes without disturbing the fillets.

4. Use a metal spatula to flip the fillets to their other side. Cook for two minutes more.

5. Place the skillet in the oven to finish cooking. Cooking time options are: 3 minutes for rare; 5 minutes for medium rare; 6 minutes for medium to well done.

TO ASSEMBLE THE SALMON

1. Rinse the serving bowls in very hot water to take the chill off. Take 2 heaping tablespoons of the hot Cauliflower Purée and smear it up the left side of the bowl.

2. Take 2 heaping tablespoons of the hot Pea Purée and smear it up the right side of bowl.

3. Place a salmon fillet in the middle of each bowl. Garnish with the Spicy Mango Salsa and lemon slices. Drizzle small amounts of avocado oil all around the dish (refer to the photo) and add edible flowers.

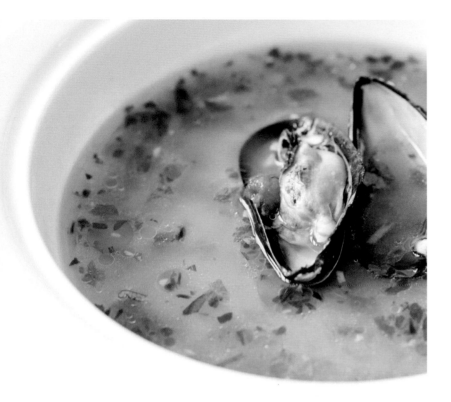

Steamed Baby Mussels in Garlic White Wine Broth

Mussels have the most impressive nutritional profile of all shellfish. They contain high levels of highly desirable long-chain fatty acids and DHA. These fats have many benefits, including improving brain function and reducing inflammatory conditions. Mussels are also a brilliant source of vitamins plus they give you a shot of important minerals such as zinc, which helps build immunity. Mussels even contain levels of iron and folic acid that rival red meats.

In a single serving, you get more than the daily dietary allowance of vitamin B_{12}. This is important to your body because it is needed to make red blood cells and is a vital part of many chemicals found in every cell.

A helpful hint when buying mussels is to make sure that they are alive prior to cooking. Shells should be tightly closed and responsive to tapping if slightly opened.

Have a soup spoon ready on the side because you are going to want to enjoy the perfectly seasoned broth the mussels have been steaming in!

SERVES 4 TO 5

INGREDIENTS

¼ cup extra-virgin olive oil

1 shallot, peeled and finely diced

4 cloves garlic, peeled and finely diced

1 teaspoon crushed red pepper

1 cup dry white wine

5 Roma tomatoes, seeded and chopped small

½ teaspoon kosher salt

1 8-ounce bottle clam juice

1 tablespoon saffron threads

4 dozen small (not large) mussels, scrubbed well and beards removed

½ cup finely chopped Italian (flat leaf) parsley

1 loaf sourdough bread

INSTRUCTIONS

1. Preheat the oven to 300F°. Place the bread in the oven and turn it off.

2. In a heavy stockpot, heat the olive oil on medium-high heat until it begins to shimmer, about 2 minutes. Add the shallot, garlic, and crushed red pepper. Lower the heat to medium and cook 5 minutes. Add the wine and cook down by half.

3. Add the tomatoes and salt; simmer 5 minutes. Add the clam juice and saffron; boil gently for 5 more minutes. Add the mussels and cover with a lid. Cook until mussels are open wide, about 5 minutes.

4. Discard any mussels that haven't opened. Sprinkle parsley over the mussels and serve immediately with the crusty bread from the oven!

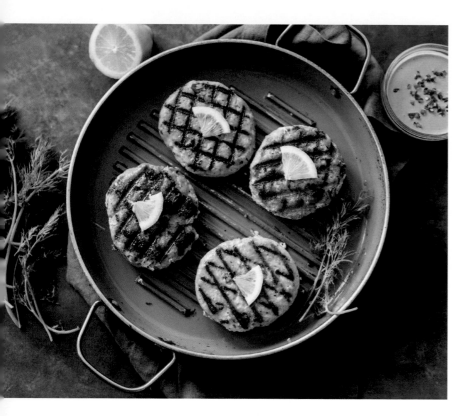

Big Omega Salmon Burgers

SERVES 4

INGREDIENTS

1 pound salmon, deboned, skin removed, and chopped into small pieces

¾ cup mayonnaise

1 cup Panko breadcrumbs

½ cup finely chopped celery

½ medium red bell pepper, seeded and chopped small

¼ cup finely diced white onion

2 scallions, white and light green parts, finely diced

2 jalapeños chiles, one diced small, one sliced into rounds

1 tablespoon chives, finely chopped

2 tablespoons Sriracha hot sauce, plus more for topping

½ cup fresh lemon juice

1 tablespoon low-sodium soy sauce

7 tablespoons extra-virgin olive oil, divided

Pinch each of kosher salt and cracked black pepper

4 whole-wheat sesame seed hamburger buns

4 cups wild arugula

4 tomato slices

4 slices thinly sliced red onion, separated into rings

Bread-and-butter pickles

INSTRUCTIONS

1. Place the salmon in a food processor and pulse-chop, leaving small chunks of salmon. Do not over process or it will be a paste.

2. In a small bowl, combine the mayonnaise, bread-crumbs, celery, bell pepper, onion, scallions, 1 tablespoon diced jalapeño, chives, two tablespoons Sriracha hot sauce, lemon juice, and soy sauce. Mix well.

3. Add the salmon and, using your hands, mix to incorporate the ingredients. Form the salmon into 4 patties to fit the size of the buns, then place them on some parchment paper.

4. Using a pastry brush coat both sides of the salmon patties with olive oil. Sprinkle them with a pinch of salt and cracked pepper.

5. Preheat an indoor grill pan or cast-iron skillet on high heat for 5 minutes.

6. Grill the salmon patties 4 minutes on each side. Do not try to flip before the 4 minutes are up or they will stick. Remove from the grill. Place on a heated plate to keep warm while you grill the buns.

7. Brush the insides of the buns with olive oil and grill to lightly toast.

TO ASSEMBLE

1. For each burger, start with the bottom bun and add 1 heaping tablespoon Sriracha hot sauce, spreading to the edge. Add 1 salmon patty, a handful of arugula, 1 tomato slice, and some onion rings. Top it with the top bun.

2. Serve with extra Sriracha hot sauce on the side and bread-and-butter pickles!

Tip: This recipe calls for a generous amount of Sriracha hot sauce, both in the salmon recipe and as a topping. If you want less heat, use less Sriracha. The same goes for the jalapeño chiles.

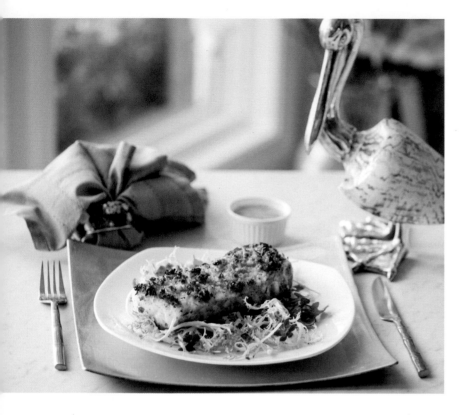

Walnut Crusted Halibut

I love fried fish with lots of tartar sauce on the side. But since I don't eat like that anymore, I wanted to come up with a coating for fish that delivers lots of flavor and a bit of a crunch but is not saturated in oil. I don't do tartar sauce, either, so I make a shallot-caper white wine sauce that delivers lots of flavor!

I use halibut for this dish. Halibut contains vitamins C, B_{12}, D, and E, and it enhances your immune system. Vitamin B_{12} protects against heart disease, cancer, stroke, and Alzheimer's.

SERVES 6

INGREDIENTS

4 tablespoons avocado oil, divided

1 tablespoon walnut oil

4 tablespoons shallots, finely chopped

⅛ teaspoon kosher salt

1 cup dry white wine

3 tablespoons fresh lemon juice

1 tablespoon unsalted butter

1 tablespoon chopped fresh dill

2 tablespoons capers

Organic coconut cooking spray

3 (6-ounce) halibut fillets, skins removed, sliced in half and refrigerated

2½ teaspoons each kosher salt and ground black pepper, divided

2 cups Panko breadcrumbs

1 cup unsalted walnuts, finely chopped

2 tablespoons Dijon mustard

½ cup freshly grated Parmesan cheese

1 tablespoon prepared horseradish

2 tablespoons chopped Italian (flat leaf) parsley

2 tablespoons lemon zest

3 tablespoon extra-virgin olive oil

4 cups loosely packed frisée lettuce

1 cup microgreens or pea shoots

Edible flowers, optional

INSTRUCTIONS

1. In a small skillet on medium heat, add 2 tablespoons avocado oil, the walnut oil, shallots, and salt. Sauté 8 minutes, until the shallots start to caramelize.

2. Turn the heat to high. Add the wine and lemon juice. Cook to reduce the liquid by almost half.

3. Reduce the heat to medium-low and stir in the butter until it has melted and the sauce has started to thicken. Remove from the heat; add the dill and capers. Set aside.

4. Preheat the oven to 425F°.

5. Generously spray a baking sheet with the coconut cooking spray.

6. Rinse the halibut and pat dry with paper towels. Season both sides with a sprinkling of salt and pepper.

7. In a shallow bowl combine the breadcrumbs, walnuts, remaining salt and pepper, Dijon mustard, Parmesan, 2 tablespoons avocado oil, horseradish, parsley, and lemon zest.

8. Roll the halibut in the breadcrumb mixture. Place the halibut pieces 1 inch apart on the baking sheet.

9. Add more breadcrumb mixture on top of each piece of fish and press it in gently. Drizzle ½ tablespoon olive oil on each piece of fish. Bake 12 to 15 minutes.

10. Garnish with the frisée lettuce, microgreens or pea shoots, and edible flowers. You can serve this dish with mashed potatoes, rice, or quinoa as a base for the fish. Serve with the shallot and caper sauce on the side!

Baked Fillet of Sole in Fresh Tomato Sauce

SERVES 6

INGREDIENTS

1 dozen small new potatoes, halved

3 tablespoons extra-virgin olive oil, divided

2½ cups of a very good jarred sauce, divided (see Tip)

2 teaspoons each of kosher salt and cracked black pepper, divided

6 (3-ounce) sole fillets

½ teaspoon crushed red pepper

1 small white onion, thinly sliced (See Chef's Note)

½ cup dry white wine

1 fennel bulb, thinly sliced

20 small Roma or cherry tomatoes, halved

20 Kalamata olives, pitted

1 lemon thinly sliced

4 sprigs fresh thyme

½ cup crumbled Greek or French feta cheese

12 basil leaves, rolled tightly and thinly sliced

½ cup Italian (flat leaf) parsley, coarsely chopped

INSTRUCTIONS

1. Preheat the oven to 400F°.

2. Bring 1 quart of water to a boil. Add the potatoes and cook 20 minutes, or until they're fork tender. Drain.

3. Coat the bottom of an ovenproof ceramic or Pyrex baking dish with 1 tablespoon olive oil (use a paper towel). Add 1 cup tomato sauce and spread evenly with a spoon to cover the entire bottom.

4. Sprinkle the salt and pepper over both sides of the sole fillets; lay over the tomato sauce. Top with the crushed red pepper, onion, wine, fennel, tomatoes, olives, potatoes, lemon, thyme, and 2 tablespoons olive oil. Pour the remaining tomato sauce over the fish. Bake 6 minutes.

5. Take the fish out of the oven and turn the broiler on high for 1 minute.

6. Place the fish under the broiler 4 inches from the heat source for 1 to 2 minutes to slightly crust the top. Do *not* leave the oven. Watch carefully so it doesn't burn; it can turn suddenly.

7. Sprinkle the feta, basil, and parsley over top.

Tip: My favorite sauce is Rao's Tomato Basil. Or you can use my homemade Roma Tomato Sauce (see p. 132).

Chef's Note: To thinly slice vegetables, I recommend using a mandoline or chef's knife.

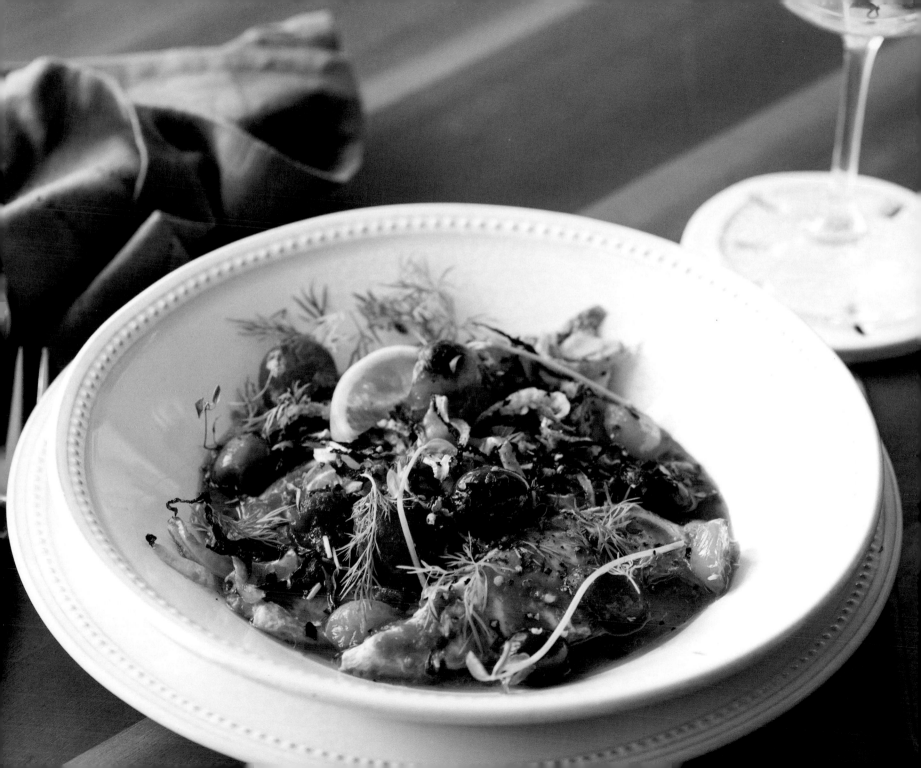

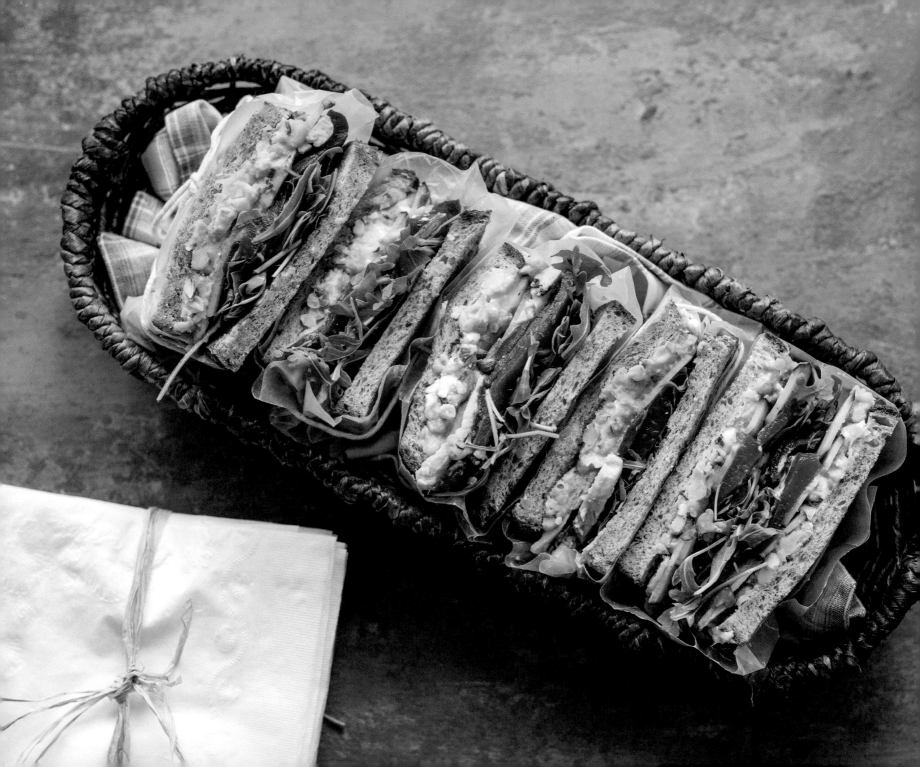

CHAPTER 8

Sandwiches

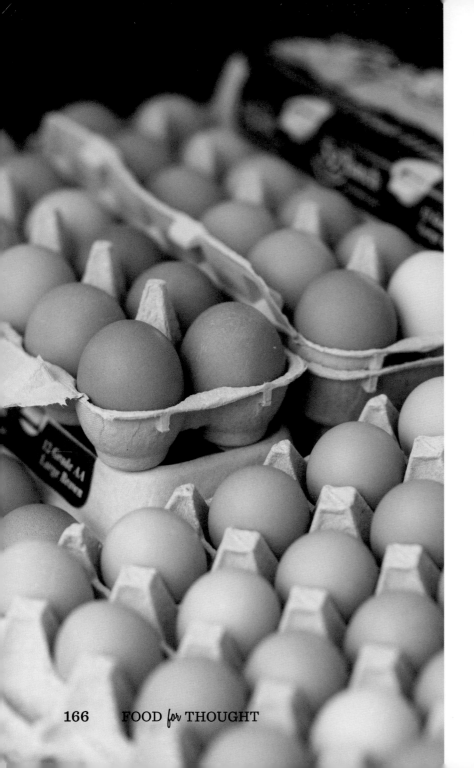

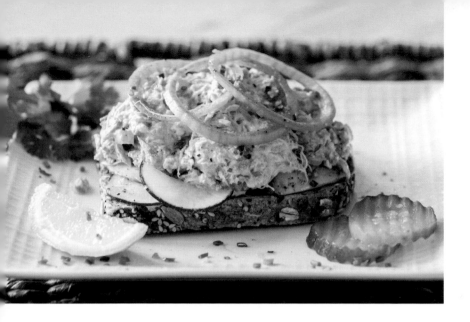

Open Face Tuna Sandwich

I prefer to use "line caught" albacore white tuna (in olive oil or water) for this sandwich. It is available in most markets and online. It is best served on multi-seeded, whole grain, whole wheat, rye, or olive bread.

SERVES 4

INGREDIENTS

2 (5-ounce) cans tuna

2 tablespoons extra-virgin olive oil

½ cup regular or vegan mayonnaise

¼ cup fresh lemon juice

1 celery rib, chopped small

1 scallion, white and light green part, finely chopped

1 tablespoon chives, finely chopped

1 tablespoon diced jalapeño with seeds, optional

½ teaspoon caraway seeds

1 tablespoon Italian (flat leaf) parsley, finely chopped

Loaf bread, sliced into 4 (½-inch) pieces

1 avocado, peeled, pitted, and halved (see Tip)

4 radishes, thinly sliced

½ red onion, thinly sliced, or 12 Pickled Onion slices (see recipe, p. 219)

2 lemons, sliced in quarters

8 bread and butter pickles

INSTRUCTIONS

1. Place the tuna in a mesh strainer and use your hands to press as much liquid out as you can. Place tuna in a bowl, add the olive oil, mayonnaise, lemon juice, celery, scallion, chopped chives, jalapeño, caraway seeds, and parsley; mix together. Cover and refrigerate for 1 hour to chill.

2. Toast the bread and place on a cutting board. Spread ¼ of the avocado over the toast, top with several slices of radish, ½ cup tuna, and 3 to 4 slices of red or pickled onions. Place the tuna sandwich on individual serving plates, and garnish with lemon slices and pickles!

3. You can also serve the tuna in a hollowed toasted whole wheat bagel.

Tip: Squeeze 1 tablespoon lemon juice on both sides of the avocado to keep it from turning brown.

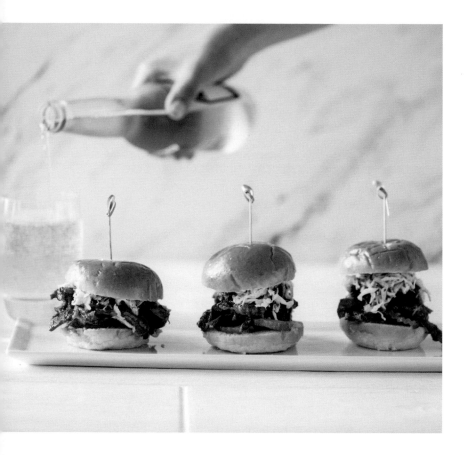

Smokin' Roasted Pulled Chicken Sliders with Slaw

I made these pulled chicken sliders for a Super Bowl party and they were a huge hit! I've been asked by my family and friends to serve them more often. I'm definitely going make these for our Fourth of July celebration because they are such a crowd-pleaser.

The chicken is slowly baked for over two hours and when it comes out of the oven it just falls off the bone. It simply melts in your mouth. The slaw gives it a clean fresh crunch and the pickles just the right amount of snappy salty brightness!

Serve up these tasty little gems with an ice-cold beer!

PULLED CHICKEN

MAKES 8 TO 10 SERVINGS

INGREDIENTS

8 (8-ounce) organic thighs, bone in, skin on

1 teaspoon Kosher salt

1 (15.5 oz.) bottle Organicville BBQ Sauce

¼ cup Sriracha hot sauce

Dill pickle slices

Whole wheat buns, 1 package (see Chef's Note)

INSTRUCTIONS FOR THE CHICKEN

1. Preheat the oven to 350F°.

2. Place the chicken thighs in a roasting pan. Sprinkle with Kosher salt.

3. Add the Sriracha hot sauce to the BBQ sauce; mix.

4. Pour the sauce over the chicken, turning to coat the bottoms of the thighs. Turn so the skin side is up. Cover with aluminum foil and roast 60 minutes. Remove the foil, turn the chicken over, and continue to roast without the foil 20 minutes.

5. Remove the chicken from the oven and let it cool.

6. Using 2 forks, pull and shred the meat from the bones.

7. Place the chicken back into the roasting pan with the barbeque sauce. Discard the skins. Save the bones to use in a stock. You can freeze them to use another time.

SLAW

INGREDIENTS

4 cups shredded green cabbage

⅓ cup mayonnaise

3 tablespoons organic apple cider vinegar

3 tablespoons fresh lemon juice

2 tablespoons seasoned rice vinegar

2 tablespoons extra-virgin olive oil

2 tablespoons Italian (flat leaf) parsley, finely chopped

1 tablespoon finely chopped jalapeño, seeded

½ teaspoon kosher salt

⅛ teaspoon cayenne pepper

INSTRUCTIONS FOR THE SLAW

1. In a large bowl combine the cabbage, mayonnaise, apple cider vinegar, lemon juice, rice wine vinegar, olive oil, parsley, jalapeño, salt, and cayenne pepper.

2. Mix well. Cover and chill in the refrigerator at least 1 hour. The slaw will keep in the refrigerator covered tightly for 2 days.

TO ASSEMBLE THE SLIDERS

1. Drain the slaw in a colander to remove excess liquid. If you don't do this the sandwich will get soggy.

2. Place 3 pickle slices on the bottom bun, add ⅓ cup pulled chicken, and top with ¼ cup or more of the slaw.

3. Secure the sandwich with a toothpick! Crack open an ice-cold beer!

Cook's Note: If you have trouble finding whole wheat "slider" buns, take regular whole wheat buns and use a 2½-inch-wide biscuit cutter to cut the wheat buns into the perfect size.

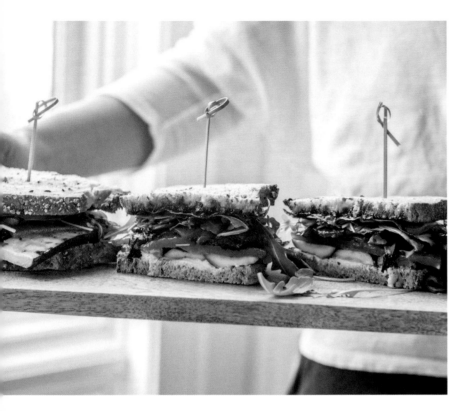

Ultimate Grilled Veggie Sandwich

To make this complete meal, I serve soup, hot or cold, to start. I love pairing this sandwich with Tomato Soup or English Spring Garden Pea Soup.

SERVES 2

INGREDIENTS

½ cup regular or vegan mayonnaise

2 tablespoons Sriracha hot sauce, plus more for topping

½ cup plus 1 tablespoon extra-virgin olive oil, divided

1 tablespoon garlic powder

1 tablespoon onion powder

1¼ teaspoon each kosher salt and ground black pepper, divided

1 medium zucchinis, sliced ¼-inch lengthwise

1 medium yellow squash, sliced ¼-inch lengthwise

1 red or yellow onion, peeled and sliced into ¼-inch rounds

2 small red bell peppers, seeded and quartered

6 (¼-inch) slices goat cheese rounds

1 tablespoon sunflower seeds

½ teaspoon crushed red pepper

8 fresh basil leaves

3 cups baby or wild arugula

1 tablespoon fresh lemon juice

4 (¼-inch) slices organic tomato

4 tablespoons cherry preserves

4 slices whole wheat ciabatta or seeded whole wheat bread in ¾-inch slices

INSTRUCTIONS

1. Mix the mayonnaise and Sriracha hot sauce. Set aside.

2. In a separate bowl, whisk together 1 tablespoon olive oil, garlic powder, onion powder, and 1 teaspoon each of salt and pepper. Using a pastry brush coat the vegetables on all sides with the olive oil mixture. Place them on a baking sheet.

3. Preheat a cast-iron indoor grill pan on high heat for 10 minutes. Starting with the zucchini and squash, grill undisturbed 4 to 5 minutes, until there is a nice char. Use a tong to flip them over and grill the other side. When they are ready, place them back on the baking sheet. Continue the process for the onion and peppers. Keep them in separate piles on the baking sheet.

TO ASSEMBLE

1. Lightly brush one side of the bread slices with the olive oil mixture. Toast (on the grill) until grill marks form, about 30 seconds.

2. For each sandwich, spread 1 heaping tablespoon Sriracha mayonnaise on the bottom slice of the grilled bread. Lay 3 goat cheese rounds and 1½ teaspoons sunflower seeds on the toasted bread. Add a pinch of crushed red pepper; gently press into the cheese. Top with 4 basil leaves.

3. Lay 3 slices each of the zucchini and squash, 2 onion rounds, and 3 to 4 quarters of red pepper.

4. In a small bowl combine the arugula, ½ cup olive oil, lemon juice, and remaining ¼ teaspoons each of salt and pepper. Mix. Add 1½ cups arugula and 2 tomato slices on each sandwich. Spread 2 tablespoons of the cherry preserves on top of each bread and place on top.

5. Slice in half diagonally using a serrated knife.

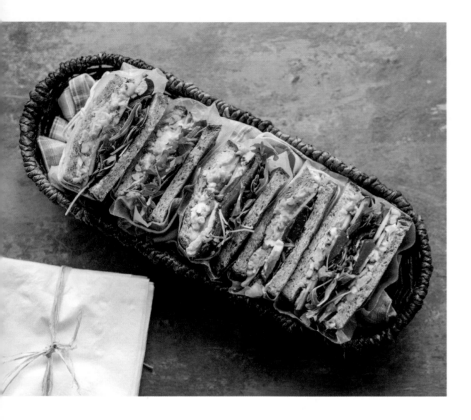

Smashed White Bean and Avocado

Protein packed, light, and a delicious choice of a sandwich for lunch! I serve these sandwiches with soup. My favorite soups to enjoy with sandwiches are the English Spring Garden Pea Soup for hot humid days, and hot Cream of Tomato Soup when it's chilly!

SERVES 4

INGREDIENTS

1 jarred red bell pepper, rinsed and patted dry

4 tablespoons extra-virgin olive oil, divided

1 garlic clove, peeled and smashed

1 (15-ounce) can white beans, drained and rinsed

¼ cup fresh lemon juice, plus 1 tablespoon

¼ teaspoon kosher salt, divided

1 teaspoon cracked black pepper

1 scallion, white and light green part, finely chopped

¼ cup Greek or French feta cheese, crumbled

2 fresh basil leaves, rolled tightly and thinly sliced

4 red onion, thinly sliced on a mandoline or with a chef's knife separated into rings

1 small cucumber, peeled, sliced thin on a mandoline or hand slicer

1 large ripe avocado, peeled, pitted and sliced into ¼-inch chunks

2 cups baby arugula

8 slices of organic whole grain, multigrain, or multi-seeded bread

INSTRUCTIONS

1. Rinse one jarred pepper with water and remove any char from the skin left on pepper. Slice into ½-inch strips and place in a small bowl with 1 tablespoon olive oil and garlic clove. Let sit for 10 minutes.

2. Combine the beans, 2 tablespoons olive oil, lemon juice, salt, pepper, and scallion. Roughly mash with a potato masher until it's chunky. Add the feta and basil; mix gently.

3. Toss the arugula with 1 tablespoon olive oil, 1 tablespoon lemon juice, and a pinch of salt.

4. Lay four slices of bread on a cutting board. Spread ½ cup of the bean mixture on each slice. Cover with 6 cucumber slices and lay several slices of the onion over the cucumbers. Add 4 slices of red bell peppers, and a handful of the tossed arugula. Split the avocado slices among the four sandwiches; press them into the top of the bread and lay it over the arugula.

5. Use your hand to gently hold the sandwich together and use a serrated knife to slice the sandwich in half. Be careful not to squish the sandwich down or the insides will come out!

Tip: Squeeze 2 tablespoons fresh lemon over the top to prevent it from turning brown.

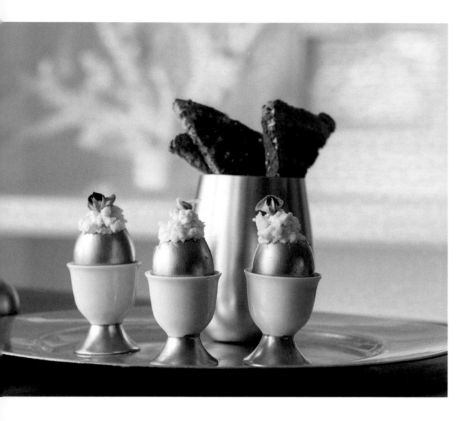

Golden Egg Salad

I love egg salad sandwiches and I wanted to come up with a different way to present them. Really—the name alone is a bit obvious and when you think about it, it doesn't really excite you all that much. So, when you see there is a recipe for egg salad sandwiches it may not excite you enough to try it.

I have always maintained that people eat with their eyes first. Presentation is everything, it excites the senses and invites you in, so, the only thing left is not to disappoint. I not only worked on presentation for this egg salad, but I worked on technique and flavors. I tested out several different variations until I came up with one I thought was just what I was looking for. This egg salad is smooth and light, with just the right amount of creaminess and a lovely tang due to the mustards I use to brighten up the flavor.

SERVES 6

INGREDIENTS

8 organic eggs (see Cook's Note)
⅓ cup regular or vegan mayonnaise
2 tablespoons Dijon mustard
1 tablespoon yellow mustard
1 celery rib, chopped small
⅛ teaspoon cayenne pepper, plus a pinch for topping
1 scallion, finely chopped
2 fresh basil leaves, finely chopped
2 tablespoons chives, finely chopped
¼ cup microgreens
Edible flowers, optional
6 pieces of toasted seeded, whole grain, or olive bread

INSTRUCTIONS

1. Place the eggs in a large saucepan and cover them with water, making sure that there is at least 2 inches of water over the eggs. Bring them to a gentle boil over high heat for 7 minutes. Remove the eggs from the heat and let them sit, covered with a lid, 7 minutes.

2. In a large bowl, prepare an ice bath of 1 quart water with 2 cups ice.

3. Remove the eggs from the saucepan with a slotted spoon and place them in the ice bath for 5 minutes. Pour out the water from the pot you cooked them in and it set aside.

4. Remove the eggs from their ice bath and place them back into the empty pot in which they were boiled. Cover with a lid and shake them back and forth, roughly 10 times, to loosen the shells. Peel them under cool running water; the shells should come off easily.

5. Slice the eggs in half and separate the yolks from the whites; place them in separate bowls. Chop the egg whites into small pieces.

6. Use a fork to finely mash the yolks. Add the mayonnaise, Dijon mustard, and yellow mustard. Mix until it's smooth and creamy. Add the chopped egg whites, celery, cayenne, scallion, basil, and chives. Mix well.

7. Cover and refrigerate for 1 hour.

8. Toast the bread, slice it into thirds, and arrange the pieces in a large glass or cup.

9. Fill each egg holder to the brim, and then some, with egg salad. Top with microgreens or edible flowers, and a pinch of cayenne.

Cook's Note: Use eggs that are at least 3 to 4 days old; the shells will peel off easier.

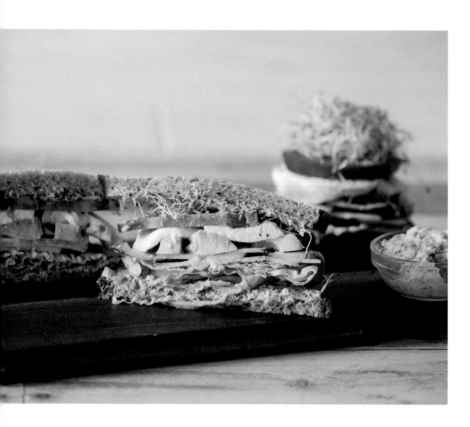

Green Sandwich

SERVES 4

8 slices whole wheat or multigrain bread

2 small ripe avocados, peeled, pitted, and halved

8 slices buffalo mozzarella, divided

1 medium to large heirloom tomato (preferably green if you can find it), sliced ¼-inch thick

Pinch kosher salt

1 cucumber with skin, thinly sliced

Handful of broccoli sprouts or microgreens

1 head butter lettuce, gently rinsed and spun dry

Green Mayo (see recipe, opposite)

Pickled Onions (see recipe, opposite)

INSTRUCTIONS FOR THE SANDWICH

1. For each sandwich, lightly toast 2 slices of bread.

2. Spread 1 heaping tablespoon of the Green Mayo on each piece. Top the bottom slice of toast with an avocado half, a pinch of salt, 2 slices mozzarella, a tomato slice, several cucumber slices, pickled onions, a handful of sprouts or microgreens, and 3 to 4 butter lettuce leaves.

3. Slice in half with a serrated knife and wrap in parchment or wax paper sandwich holder.

GREEN MAYO

INGREDIENTS

½ cup basil leaves

¼ cup tarragon leaves

1 small clove garlic

⅓ cup chives, finely chopped

2 anchovy fillets

1 tablespoon lime zest

¼ teaspoon salt

⅓ cup mayonnaise

3 tablespoons fresh lemon juice

INSTRUCTIONS

In a food processor add the basil, tarragon, garlic, chives, anchovies, lime zest, salt, and mayonnaise. Purée 1 minute; add the lemon juice. Pour into a glass bowl, cover, and refrigerate to chill. Green Mayo will keep for 4 to 5 days stored in the refrigerator.

PICKLED ONIONS

INGREDIENTS

2 white onions, peeled and thinly sliced

½ cup white wine vinegar

2 tablespoons monk fruit sugar

1 teaspoon kosher salt

¼ teaspoon cracked black pepper

INSTRUCTIONS

In a glass Mason jar, combine the onions, vinegar, monk fruit sweetener, salt, and pepper. Let the mixture sit at least 3 hours before using or refrigerate. It will keep in the refrigerator for up to a week.

Tip: Squeeze lemon juice over avocado halves to keep them from turning brown.

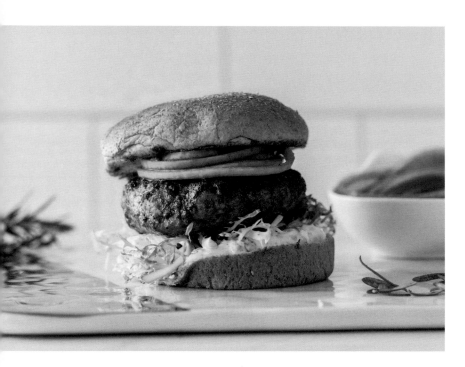

Lamb Burgers

If you use my method to cook the lamb for these burgers, it will ensure the lamb will turn out perfectly cooked—juicy and moist. Just go with it.

LAMB BURGER

SERVES 4

INGREDIENTS

1½ pounds ground lamb

1 teaspoon onion salt

1 teaspoon garlic powder

1 teaspoon kosher salt

1 tablespoon scallion, white and light green part, finely chopped

1 tablespoon Italian (flat leaf) parsley, finely chopped

1 tablespoons fresh dill, finely chopped

1 tablespoon fresh mint, finely chopped

2 tablespoons regular or vegan mayonnaise

1 egg yolk

½ cup Panko breadcrumbs

¼ teaspoon cayenne pepper

2 tablespoons safflower oil

3 cups frisée lettuce

6 whole wheat sesame buns or olive bread sliced ¼-inch thin

Cucumber-Yogurt Sauce (see recipe, opposite)

Pickled onions or 1 red onion cut in ¼-inch slices

INSTRUCTIONS FOR BURGER

1. In a large bowl, combine the lamb, onion salt, garlic powder, salt, scallions, parsley, dill, mint, mayonnaise, egg yolk, breadcrumbs, and cayenne pepper. Using your hands, mix the ingredients well. Form four 6-ounce patties, approximately 4 inches wide and 1-inch thick.

2. Heat a heavy-bottomed skillet on high heat for 1 minute. Add 2 tablespoons safflower oil and swirl in the pan. Heat for one minute. Add the lamb. Turn the heat down to medium.

3. Cook the lamb undisturbed for 2 minutes, then flip it over and cook 2 minutes.

4. Flip it over and cook 2 minutes, then flip over again and cook another 2 minutes.

5. Repeat steps 1 and 2.

6. Cook for 3 minutes, flip again for another 3 minutes.

7. At this point the lamb will be rare to medium-rare. If you prefer the meat to be well done, cook another 3 minutes.

8. Transfer the lamb burger from the skillet onto a cutting board and let the patties rest 5 minutes.

9. Toast the buns or the olive bread lightly.

10. Lay the four bottom buns on a chopping board. Add 3 tablespoons Cucumber-Yogurt Sauce, a handful of frisée lettuce, a lamb patty, and as much pickled onion as you like.

CUCUMBER-YOGURT SAUCE

MAKES ABOUT 1½ CUPS

INGREDIENTS

1 cucumber, peeled, seeded, and chopped small
2 cups whole-milk Greek yogurt, plain
2 tablespoons extra-virgin olive oil
2 tablespoons fresh lemon juice
1 tablespoon chopped fresh dill
1 tablespoon chopped fresh mint
¼ teaspoon each kosher salt and cracked black pepper
⅛ teaspoon cayenne pepper

INSTRUCTIONS FOR SAUCE

1. Mix the cucumber, yogurt, olive oil, lemon juice, dill, mint, salt, pepper, and cayenne pepper.

2. Cover and refrigerate 1 hour to chill. Keep in the refrigerator until ready to use.

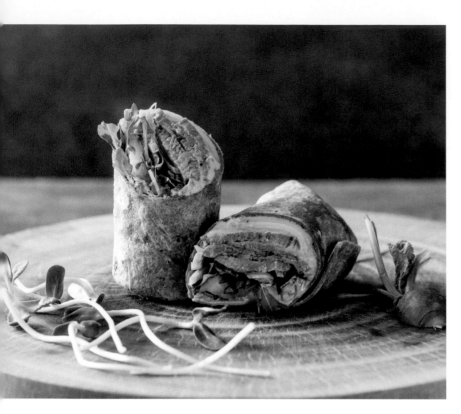

Sriracha Beef Tortilla Roll

This sandwich is for people who like a little heat! If you can't take the heat, I included an alternative marinade at the end of this recipe.

I suggest you cook the beef on an outdoor grill. If you do grill inside, make sure to turn on the exhaust vent to high and open a window. Since it is spicy, it may make you cough a bit and your eyes will water because of the heat in the Sriracha sauce. Been there, done that, but it's worth it!

SERVES 4

INGREDIENTS

3 teaspoons kosher salt

3 teaspoons garlic powder

1½ pounds flank steak

½ cup Sriracha hot sauce

¼ cup soy sauce

¼ cup extra-virgin olive oil

3 tablespoons fresh lime juice

2 garlic cloves, peeled and crushed

4 sandwich dill pickles, sliced lengthwise in ¼-inch slices

4 slices Muenster or Monterey Jack cheese, cut in half

2 cups loosely packed arugula

1 small red onion, thinly sliced

4 tablespoons Sriracha Mayo (see recipe, p. 216)

4 (8- to 10-inch) whole wheat tortillas

INSTRUCTIONS

1. Whisk the kosher salt and garlic powder. Sprinkle half of the mixture on each side of the steak.

2. In a medium bowl, whisk the Sriracha hot sauce, soy sauce, olive oil, and lime juice. Pour over the meat and turn over to coat both sides; add the garlic cloves. Cover tightly with plastic wrap and marinate for 6 hours, or overnight for the best flavor.

3. Before you grill the meat make sure you have plenty of ventilation. When you're ready to serve, heat a cast-iron indoor grill pan or heavy-duty skillet for 10 minutes. Lift the marinated flank steak with metal tongs and let as much of the marinade drip off as you can.

4. Place the flank on the grill for 2½ minutes without disturbing it. Turn the steak over and do the same with the other side. The beef will be medium-rare.

5. Remove from heat and let sit 10 minutes before slicing against the grain into thin strips.

TO ASSEMBLE

1. Make sure you leave a 1½-inch space on each side of a tortilla when adding ingredients to roll and tuck.

2. Place a tortilla on a clean chopping board. Spread 1 heaping tablespoon Sriracha mayonnaise over the whole tortilla.

3. Lay 2 half-slices of cheese on the lower third of the tortilla along with 6 to 8 strips of beef, several thin slices of onion, ½ cup arugula, and 1 dill pickle slice.

4. Roll over tightly twice, fold over the sides of tortilla, and tuck it in. Continue rolling to form a cylinder. Use a serrated knife to slice on the diagonal.

ALTERNATE FLANK STEAK MARINADE

For a milder marinade, use this recipe on the flank steak to make your sandwich.

1½ pounds flank steak
4 tablespoons extra-virgin olive oil
½ cup tamari (gluten-free soy sauce)
1 tablespoon ground cumin
2 teaspoons coriander
2 teaspoons chili oil
4 tablespoons fresh lime juice
2 garlic cloves, smashed and peeled
½ teaspoon kosher salt

INSTRUCTIONS FOR THE MARINADE

1. Place the steak in a glass dish large enough to hold all the pieces flat.

2. In a glass bowl, whisk the olive oil, soy sauce, cumin, coriander, chili oil, and lime juice. Add the garlic. Pour the marinade over the steak. Cover and marinate in the refrigerator overnight.

3. When you are ready to grill remove the steak from the refrigerator and let stand at room temperature for 30 minutes.

4. Follow the grilling instructions from the first recipe.

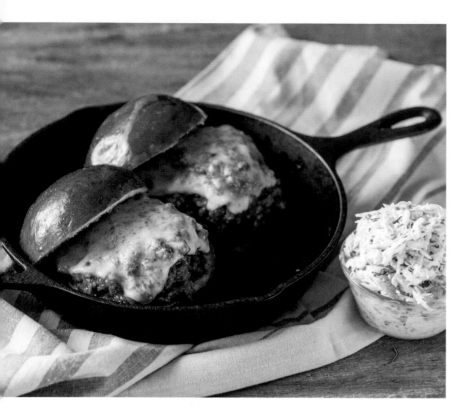

Sloppy Joes

SERVES 4

INGREDIENTS

3 tablespoons safflower oil

1 medium onion, minced

4 scallions, white and light green parts, finely chopped

1 tablespoon ground cumin

1 teaspoon onion powder

1 teaspoon garlic powder

½ teaspoon each kosher salt and cracked black pepper

1 pound ground dark turkey meat

2 turkey sausages, casings removed

½ cup tomato ketchup

1 cup canned black beans, drained and rinsed

2 tablespoons minced chipotle chili in adobo sauce

2 tablespoons jalapeño, seeded, finely chopped

½ teaspoon Stevia

1 tablespoon Dijon mustard

⅓ cup water

4 slices Monterey Jack Cheese

4 whole wheat seeded buns

Coleslaw (see recipe, opposite)

Dill pickles

INSTRUCTIONS

1. Line a baking sheet with parchment paper.

2. Heat a cast-iron skillet for one minute. Add the oil, onions, and scallions. Sauté 3 to 5 minutes. Add the cumin, onion powder, garlic powder, salt, and pepper. Mix well and cook 3 minutes, stirring constantly.

3. Add the turkey and turkey sausages; use a metal spatula to break the meat into small pieces. Sauté 10 to 12 minutes or until the turkey starts to caramelize. Stir in ketchup, and mix, Add the beans, chipotle chili, jalapeño, Stevia, and Dijon mustard. Stir. Add the water and cook down for 5 minutes.

4. Set the broiler to High.

5. Pull out some bread from the middle of the bottom and top buns to make a small cradle to hold the meat.

6. Place the four bottom buns on the baking sheet lined with parchment paper.

7. Spoon 1 cup turkey meat onto the bottom buns; top each with a slice of cheese. Broil until the cheese has melted, usually 1 minute. When the cheese has melted, remove the buns from broiler.

8. Top with a nice helping of slaw and then the top of the bun. Add dill pickles on the side!

Tip: Do not walk away from the oven while melting the cheese on the buns. It can burn super-fast, so watch it carefully.

COLESLAW

INGREDIENTS

1 pound green cabbage, shredded

$\frac{1}{3}$ cup regular or vegan mayonnaise

2 tablespoons apple cider vinegar

2 tablespoons extra-virgin olive oil

2 tablespoons Italian (flat leaf) parsley, coarsely chopped

$\frac{1}{2}$ cup shredded carrots

2 scallions, white and light green parts, finely chopped

1 jalapeño, seeded, finely chopped

1 teaspoon kosher salt

$\frac{1}{8}$ teaspoon cayenne pepper

$\frac{1}{2}$ cup Virginia peanuts

INSTRUCTIONS

1. Combine the cabbage, mayonnaise, vinegar, olive oil, parsley, carrots, scallions, jalapeño, salt, pepper, cayenne, and peanuts into a medium-sized bowl. Mix well.

2. Cover and refrigerate until ready to serve.

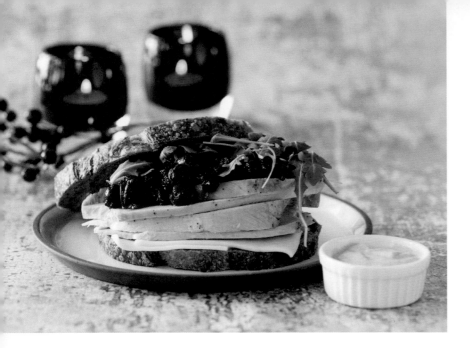

Savory Roasted Turkey Sandwiches with Cranberry Sauce

I love this cranberry sauce! The spices are a perfectly paired with the turkey, pears, and other ingredients. The tart flavor of the cranberries gives a turkey sandwich that could be bland, the kick it needs to send it over the top!

Cranberries are available fresh from mid-September to December. When they are out of season, I use organic frozen cranberries.

You can make the cranberry sauce and the Dijon Mayo up to 3 days before and store in an airtight container in the refrigerator.

CRANBERRY SAUCE

MAKES 8 TO 10 SERVINGS

INGREDIENTS

1 (12-ounce) bag fresh cranberries

1 cup fresh orange juice

½ cup monk fruit sweetener

1 tablespoon pure maple syrup

1 teaspoon ground cinnamon

1 tablespoon orange zest

1 tablespoon port wine

¼ cup chopped walnuts, toasted

2 tablespoons coarsely chopped fresh mint

INSTRUCTIONS

1. Place the cranberries, orange juice, monk fruit, maple syrup, cinnamon, orange zest, and port wine into a medium saucepan over high heat. Bring to a boil. When the cranberries begin to pop open, boil 3 to 5 minutes longer. Turn off the heat and let cool to room temperature.

2. Refrigerate 2 hours, or overnight to thoroughly chill. Just before serving add the walnuts and mint. You will have leftover cranberry sauce, which you can use for desserts or more sandwiches!

DIJON MAYO

INGREDIENTS

3 heaping tablespoons Dijon mustard

1½ cups regular or vegan mayonnaise

¼ teaspoon cayenne pepper

1 tablespoon Tabasco

1 tablespoon lemon juice

INSTRUCTIONS

Whisk the Dijon mustard, mayonnaise, cayenne pepper, Tabasco, and lemon juice. Set aside.

TURKEY SANDWICH

SERVES 4

INGREDIENTS

2 cups baby spinach leaves

2 cups baby or wild arugula

1 tablespoon extra-virgin olive

1 tablespoon fresh lemon juice

Pinch of Kosher salt

8 slices whole grain or heavy seeded grain bread

1 avocado peeled, pitted, cut into ¼-inch slices (see Tip)

8 slices Havarti cheese

10 to 12 thin slices roasted turkey breast.

2 ripe pears, peeled, cored, and sliced into ¼-inch pieces (see Tip)

Cranberry Sauce (see recipe, opposite)

8 tablespoons Dijon Mayonnaise (see recipe, above)

INSTRUCTIONS

1. Toss the spinach and arugula with the olive oil, lemon juice, and salt.

2. For each sandwich lay 4 slices of bread on a cutting board and spread 2 tablespoons Dijon Mayonnaise on each.

3. Add ¼ of the avocado, plus 1 slice of cheese.

4. Lay 3 to 4 slices turkey, 4 pear slices per sandwich, and a handful of the tossed spinach-arugula mix.

5. Top with 2 to 3 tablespoons Cranberry Sauce. Add another dollop of Dijon Mayonnaise on the top piece of bread. Place on top of sandwich and hold down each sandwich firmly, slice in half with a serrated knife, and serve!

6. Serve any extra Dijon Mayonnaise on the side.

Tip: To keep the avocado from turning brown, squeeze 1 tablespoon of lemon juice over it. For the pears, squeeze 2 tablespoons of lemon juice over them.

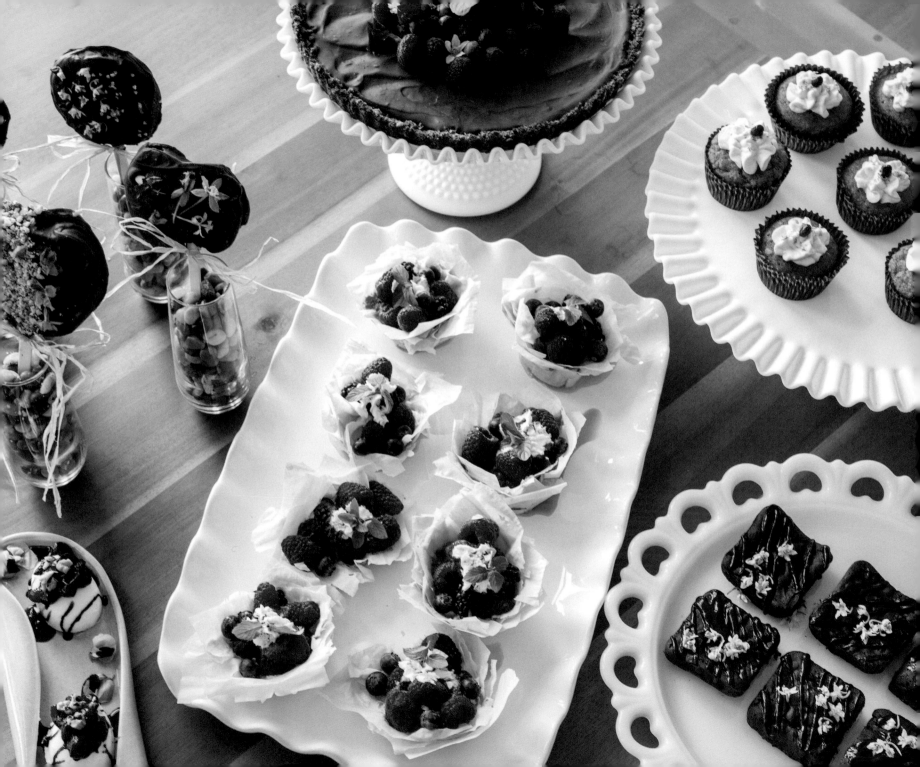

CHAPTER 9

Desserts

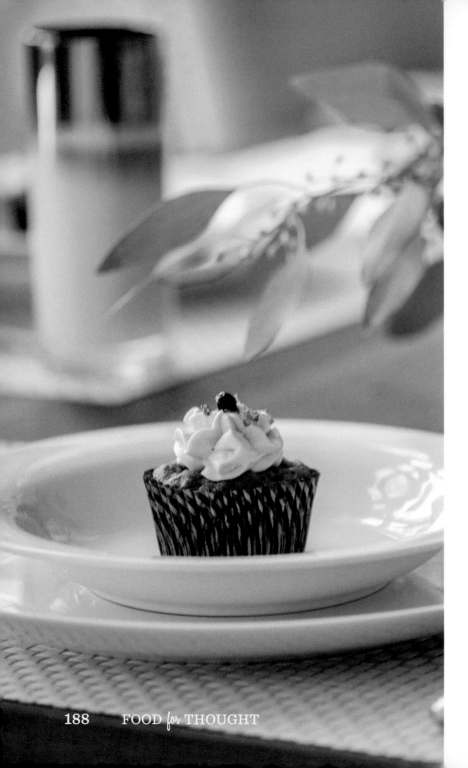

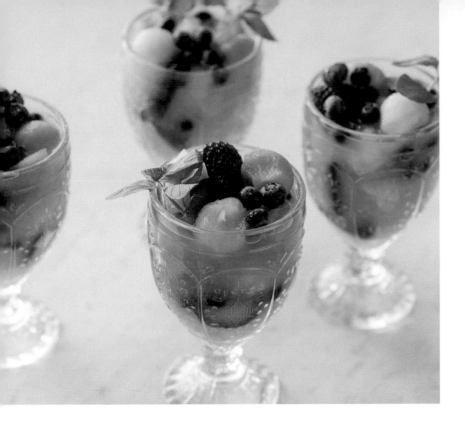

Fresh Fruit

Sometimes I like to finish a light dinner such as grilled chicken, fish, or even a sandwich with a chilled cup of seasonal fresh fruit. I used in-season melons, strawberries, and blueberries with freshly squeezed orange juice. You can pick any fruit you like to make yours. I also serve them for breakfast and for a pick-me-up snack in the afternoon! Or pair it with a lovely chilled Riesling for a refreshing way to finish a main meal.

SERVES 6

INGREDIENTS

1 small cantaloupe, seeded

1 honeydew or casaba melon, seeded

1 pint strawberries, hulled

½ cup blueberries

4 cups fresh orange juice

1 bunch fresh mint

INSTRUCTIONS

1. Use a melon baller to make small balls of the cantaloupe and honeydew. Alternate the melon balls with the strawberries and blueberries among the serving glasses or bowls.

2. Add a splash of the orange juice to each, and garnish with mint.

Tip: A 4-ounce serving (about 1 cup) is the perfect amount.

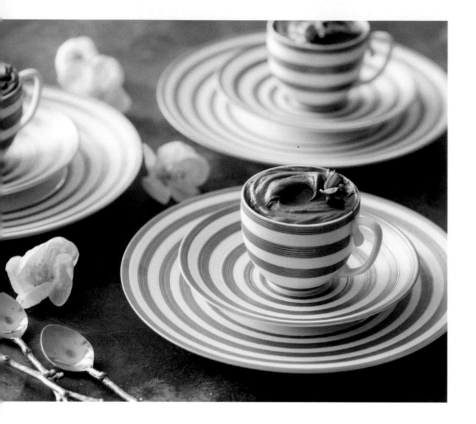

Chocolate Mousse—No Dairy, No Processed Sugar, No Kidding!

This Chocolate Mousse is an extremely creamy and satisfying dessert. I guarantee you won't feel guilty or have a tummy ache from processed sugar or dairy products because there are none in this mousse. Whoever thought a dessert would actually be good for your health? But it is! The main ingredient is sweet potato and in one medium spud there is over 400 percent of your daily requirement of vitamin A. They contain high amounts of fiber and potassium, and are low in calories.

When I serve this chocolate mousse, I tell my guests up front that there is no dairy or processed sugar in the dessert and that it is made with a secret ingredient. They all try to figure it out, and avocado is the food that is mentioned most frequently. They are really surprised when I tell them it's actually a sweet potato!

MAKES 12 TO 14 (3-OUNCE) SERVINGS

INGREDIENTS

1 cup hazelnut milk

1 cup organic chocolate chips

2 (1 pound) sweet potatoes, not the orange colored, peeled and cut into 1½-inch rounds

2 teaspoons kosher salt

¼ cup pure maple syrup

1 tablespoon vanilla extract

2 tablespoons safflower oil

¼ cup organic smooth peanut butter

¼ cup (2 ounces) espresso coffee

Non-dairy whipped coconut cream

Fresh mint, coarsely chopped

¼ cup Toasted Walnuts (see recipe, p. 221)

1 cup fresh raspberries

1 cup Toasted Coconut (see recipe, p. 221), optional

INSTRUCTIONS

1. Pour the chocolate chips into a double boiler over simmering water. Add the hazelnut milk. Use a wooden spoon to mix the chocolate chips and milk together until the chocolate has melted. Turn off the heat, and cover with a lid.

2. Steam the sweet potatoes for 30 minutes or until soft. Use a paring knife to check for doneness; if the knife slides in and out easily, they are ready.

3. Place the cooked sweet potatoes into a blender, add the melted chocolate mixture. Turn the blender on, and through the feed tube add the salt, maple syrup, vanilla extract, safflower oil, peanut butter, and espresso. Blend 1 minute on high speed until the mixture is smooth and creamy.

4. Pour mixture into a bowl and cover with plastic wrap. Refrigerate 3 hours to chill.

TO SERVE

Place ½ cup dry measuring cup serving in a dessert bowl or dessert glass and garnish with the whipped coconut cream, walnuts, raspberries, and toasted coconut, if desired.

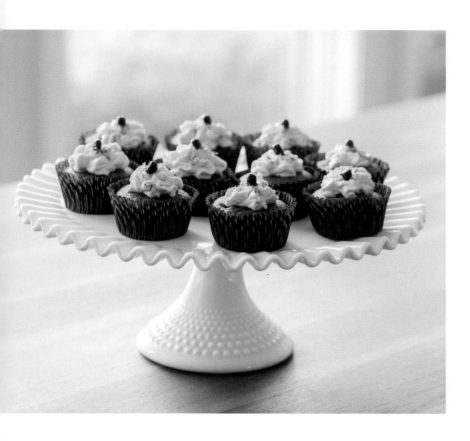

Pumpkin Cupcakes with Cream Cheese Frosting

Frankly, I was shocked when I made these cupcakes for the first time. It took several tries, and to be honest, I was skeptical. When it comes to baking—unless you used butter, sugar, and white flour—a cupcake wasn't going to bake up nice and moist, or taste good.

I was wrong. After a few misses, I finally found the perfect combination of ingredients and baking time and they turned out simply delicious. They are light, definitely moist, and filled with ingredients that are good for you. The cream cheese frosting puts this dessert over the top. Just a dollop of pure creamy goodness adds the right amount of total satisfaction!

I personally love to enjoy this cupcake with a cup of hot tea!

MAKES 12 CUPCAKES

INGREDIENTS

¾ cup organic unbleached flour

¼ cup whole flaxseeds

1 teaspoon ground cinnamon

1 teaspoon ground ginger

½ teaspoon grated nutmeg

⅛ teaspoon ground cloves

1 teaspoon baking soda

¼ teaspoon salt

2 eggs, lightly beaten

¾ cup plain canned pumpkin (not pie filling)

⅔ cup maple syrup

¼ cup safflower oil

INSTRUCTIONS

1. Preheat the oven to 350F°.

2. Line a 12-cupcake baking tin with cupcake papers.

3. Whisk the flour, flaxseeds, cinnamon, ginger, nutmeg, cloves, baking soda, and salt.

4. In a separate bowl, whisk the eggs, pumpkin, maple syrup, and safflower oil until well combined. Add the flour mixture to the pumpkin mixture, and fold until any flour streaks are gone. Do not overmix.

5. Spoon the batter into cupcake liners until each liner is three-fourths full.

6. Bake 18 minutes or until a toothpick comes out slightly moist.

7. Remove the cupcakes from the oven and cool in the tin for 5 minutes. Lift the cupcakes gently out of the tin and place them on a wire baking rack to cool for an hour.

CREAM CHEESE FROSTING

MAKES 2 CUPS

INGREDIENTS

8 ounces reduced-fat cream cheese, at room temperature

1 tablespoon fresh lemon juice

2 tablespoons coconut butter

1 tablespoon vanilla extract

1 tablespoon lime zest

2 tablespoons pomegranate seeds

INSTRUCTIONS

1. In a mixer or food processor, combine the cream cheese, lemon juice, coconut butter, and vanilla extract. Process on medium-high until the frosting is smooth and creamy.

2. Place the frosting into a piping bag with a #2 tip and squeeze a dollop on the top of each cupcake. Sprinkle the cupcakes with the lime zest and add a few pomegranate seeds on the top of each one!

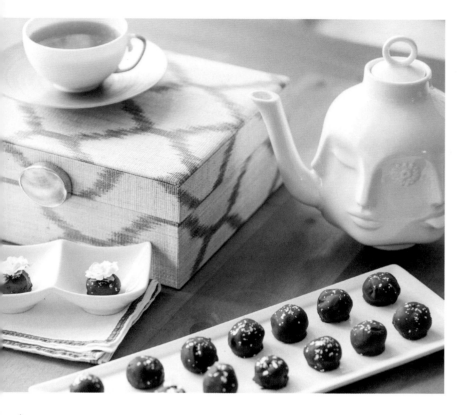

Peanut Butter Amazeballs

I am an insane lover of peanut butter and chocolate together, as you probably can guess by now. I came up with these heavenly peanut butter balls that I have dubbed "Amazeballs!" The ratio of chocolate to peanut butter is perfect, the recipe contains pure natural ingredients, and each one is just the right portion size. Because they are all natural and easy to digest, I enjoy two as a pick-me-up in the afternoon with hot tea!

MAKES 4 DOZEN

INGREDIENTS

1 cup 100% organic natural crunchy peanut butter

4 tablespoons pure maple syrup

¼ teaspoon kosher salt

3 tablespoons coconut flour

1 cup dark chocolate chips

2 teaspoons coconut oil

¼ cup pomegranate seeds

Edible gold leaf, available online

Any type of chopped nuts, optional

INSTRUCTIONS

1. Line a baking sheet with parchment paper.

2. Chances are the peanut butter will have to be stirred together to incorporate the oil that has risen to the top of the jar. When it is smooth and creamy, it is ready to use.

3. In a bowl, add the peanut butter and maple syrup, and whisk together until it is thick. Add the coconut flour and mix well. Let the peanut better sit for 10 minutes.

4. Roll into ¼ oz. balls (size of a large grape) and place them on the baking sheet.

5. Combine the chocolate chips and coconut oil in a double boiler and melt, whisking until smooth. Cool for 15 minutes.

6. Dip and roll the balls into the melted chocolate with a fork.

7. Lift them gently and tap against the side of the bowl to let any excess chocolate run off.

8. Use a second fork to push the balls onto the parchment paper. Continue the process until all of the balls are covered in chocolate. When all the balls are done, add several tiny pieces of the edible gold leaf and one pomegranate seed on the top of each one.

9. You can also sprinkle chopped nuts over the top while they are still wet.

10. Place in the refrigerator to firm up for 1 hour. They will keep in the refrigerator for up to a week in an airtight container. They are delicious served cold, frozen, or room temperature.

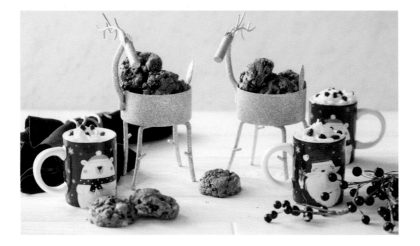

Chocolate Chip Scoopers

MAKES 2 DOZEN

INGREDIENTS

1½ cups oat flour

1 teaspoon baking soda

1 teaspoon cinnamon

½ teaspoon kosher salt

¼ cup coconut oil

¼ cup unsalted butter, melted

1 tablespoon pure vanilla extract

1 large egg

4 tablespoons dark brown monk fruit sweetener

1½ cups dark chocolate chips

½ cup raisins

¼ cup chopped hazelnuts or walnuts

INSTRUCTIONS

1. Preheat the oven to 325F°.

2. Line a cookie sheet with parchment paper.

3. Place the oat flour in a blender and process until it resembles a flour or powder.

4. In a mixer fitted with a paddle, beat the coconut oil, butter, vanilla extract, egg, and dark brown monk fruit sweetener together until incorporated.

5. In separate bowl, whisk the oat flour, baking soda, cinnamon, and salt.

6. Combine the oat flour mixture and the egg mixture; turn the mixer on medium to mix thoroughly. Add the chocolate chips, raisins, and nuts. Mix until combined.

7. Chill the dough for 1 hour in the refrigerator. Use a small ice cream scoop or a tablespoon to drop heaping helpings of the dough onto the lined cookie sheet 2 inches apart.

8. Bake 10 to 12 minutes until the cookies are lightly browned around the edges and slightly soft in the middle.

9. Remove the baking sheet from the oven and use a metal spatula to gently lift the cookies and place them on a cooling rack for 30 minutes.

10. The chocolate will be soft and melty and the cookie will be extremely fragile. They may crumble a bit at this point but will harden as they cool. Store in a cool place. These cookies taste even better the next day!

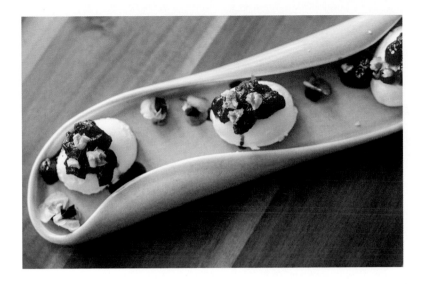

Coconut Dairy-Free Ice Cream with Cinnamon Spice Cranberry Sauce

When I made this recipe for cranberry sauce the first time, I thought it would work well both with the Thanksgiving meal, and double as a dessert! I tried it over dairy-free ice cream and everyone loved it. It is so refreshing and different. Try it over frozen yogurt, too, and don't forget a squiggle of chocolate sauce! So good!

SERVES 4

INGREDIENTS

1 (12-ounce) bag fresh cranberries

1 cup fresh orange juice

½ cup monk fruit sweetener

¼ cup port wine

1 teaspoon ground cinnamon

1 tablespoon orange zest

¼ cup chopped walnuts, toasted

¼ cup coarsely chopped fresh mint

Organic chocolate sauce, store-bought

INSTRUCTIONS

1. Place the cranberries, orange juice, monk fruit, port wine, and cinnamon into a medium saucepan. Bring to a boil. When the cranberries begin to pop open, boil 3 to 5 minutes longer. Turn off the heat and let it cool to room temperature.

2. Cool in the refrigerator 2 hours or overnight. Just before serving, add the orange zest, walnuts, and mint.

3. For dessert, just spoon the cranberries over your choice of dairy-free coconut ice cream, an alternate dairy-free ice cream, or a sugar-free sorbet.

4. Don't forget the squiggle of chocolate sauce over the top!

Tip: Fresh cranberries are available September through December. Use organic frozen cranberries if out of season.

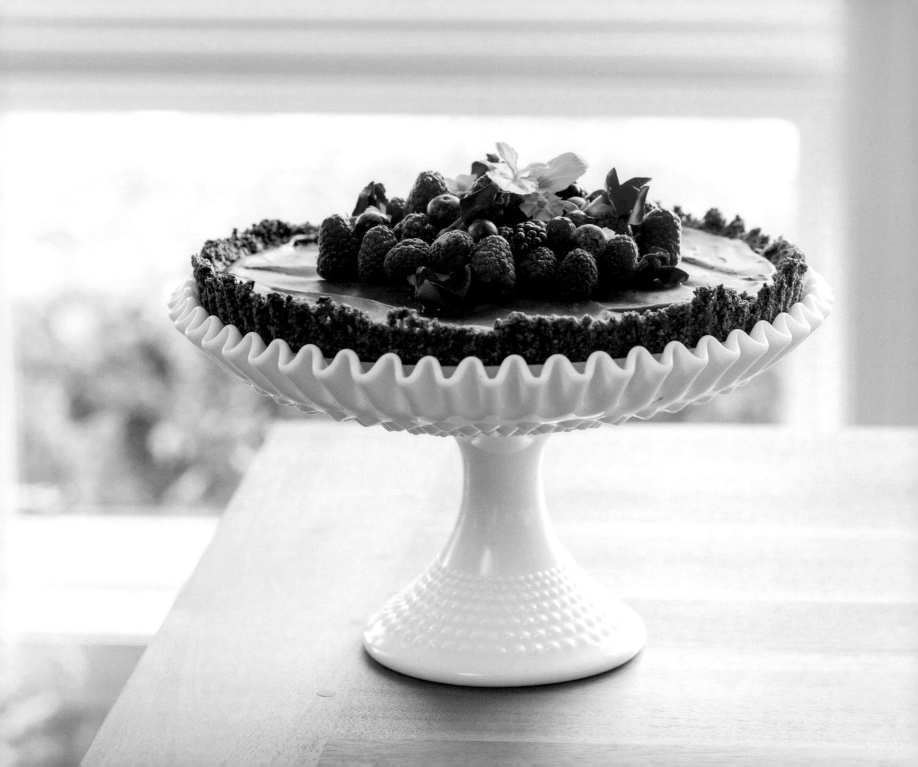

Ganache Tart with Coconut Crust

MAKES 14 TO 16 SLICES

GANACHE TART

INGREDIENTS

2 cups coconut cream

1 teaspoon pure vanilla extract

1 tablespoon maple syrup

5 ounces bittersweet chocolate, 85–90% cacao, chopped into small pieces

1 teaspoon salt

INSTRUCTIONS

1. Heat the coconut cream, vanilla extract, and maple syrup in a saucepan to a gentle boil. Turn the heat off and let sit, covered, 10 minutes. Whisk in the chocolate and salt until smooth.

2. Pour the chocolate ganache into the tart shell and refrigerate 2 hours until the ganache sets. Garnish with the pinch of coarse sea salt, the fresh berries, and edible flowers.

3. Slice into small portions; a little goes a long way!

COCONUT CRUST

INGREDIENTS

⅓ cup coconut oil

¼ cup brown rice syrup

2 cups shredded coconut

1 tablespoon raw cacao powder

INSTRUCTIONS

1. Preheat the oven to 350F°.

2. Melt coconut oil and brown rice syrup in a saucepan. Remove from the heat and add the shredded coconut and cacao powder. Mix well.

3. Press the mixture into the bottom and ¼ inch up the sides of a tart pan. Bake 15 to 20 minutes. Remove the tart from the oven and set aside to cool 15 minutes.

GARNISH

INGREDIENTS

⅛ teaspoon coarse sea salt

½ cup fresh raspberries

½ cup fresh blackberries

Edible flower petals, available online (optional)

INSTRUCTIONS

Arrange the above items on top of the tart using your own design or follow mine!

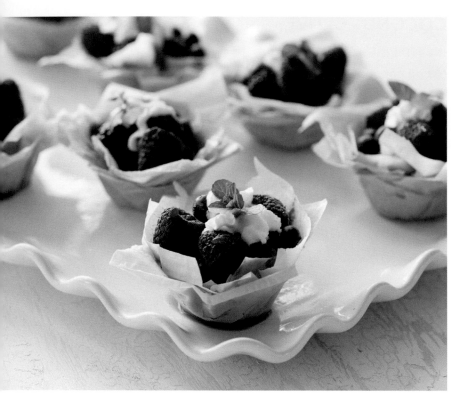

Phyllo Cups with Greek Yogurt, Berries, and Honey

There are so many yogurts available, but I'm not a fan of fruit-flavored yogurts or fruit-on-the-bottom yogurts; they have so much sugar added to them. I prefer Greek-style yogurt. The liquid whey is strained out, making it thicker and creamier, and it doesn't have the tart taste that regular yogurt has.

If you want to make your own Greek-style yogurt, you can easily do it. Just pour plain yogurt into a cheesecloth-lined strainer positioned over a bowl to catch the liquid. It usually takes 2 hours to make 2 quarts of plain yogurt.

All yogurts are an excellent source of calcium, potassium, protein, zinc, vitamins B_6 and B_{12}, and probiotics. Probiotics work by changing the balance of bacteria in your gut. We now know gut bacteria has been linked to improved digestion, enhanced immune function, and reduced risk of many diseases. Please take the time to check the label and make sure it says "contains live and active cultures."

MAKES 12 CUPS

INGREDIENTS

2 pints fresh raspberries

½ teaspoon Stevia

2 tablespoons lemon juice

Coconut cooking spray

1 (3½-ounce) package phyllo dough

3 cups plain Greek yogurt

2 cups raspberries

1 cup blueberries

3 tablespoons lemon juice

1 tablespoon ground cinnamon

3 tablespoons chopped walnuts

½ cup coarsely chopped fresh mint leaves

INSTRUCTIONS

1. Combine the raspberries, Stevia and lemon juice in a food processor or blender. Blend 1 minute. Press the mixture through a fine mesh strainer to remove all the seeds. Pour into a needle-nose plastic bottle and refrigerate until ready to use. The raspberry syrup will keep 3 days in the refrigerator.

2. When you're ready to serve, preheat the oven to 350F°.

3. Spray two 12-cup muffin tins generously with cooking spray. Remove 6 phyllo sheets from the package. Lay them on a cutting board and cover with a slightly damp kitchen towel to keep them from drying out.

4. Lay 1 sheet of phyllo dough on a work surface, and spray lightly with cooking spray. Slice the sheet into approximately 6 x 6-inch squares. Place 1 square inside each muffin cup and press the bottom to fit into the cup.

5. Repeat the process, laying the other 4 squares at different angles until all 5 have been gently pressed in. The ends of the phyllo dough will be taller than the cups and overlap so you won't be able to lay the phyllo cups right next to each other.

6. Skip the next cup in the tin, leaving it empty, and go to the next one. Repeat the process of laying the phyllo for the rest of the cups until you have a dozen cups.

7. Bake 8 minutes or until golden brown. Remove from the oven and cool 30 minutes. Gently lift the phyllo cups and place them on a platter or individual dessert plates.

8. Fill each cup with 2 tablespoons yogurt. Divide the berries between each cup, and top with 1 tablespoon raspberry syrup. Add a pinch of cinnamon, a teaspoon or more of walnuts, and the mint. Serve immediately.

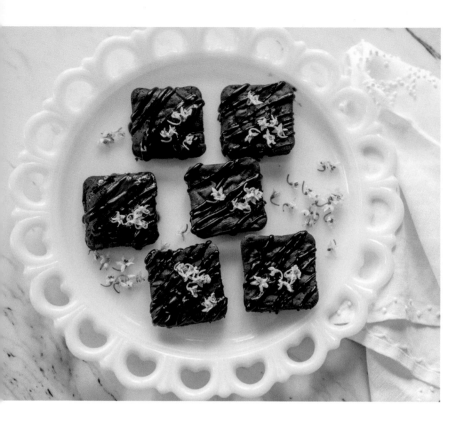

Brownies

These brownies deliver all that and more. They have a rich chocolate flavor that's sure to please any chocolate lover. The best part is, I can enjoy a dessert that doesn't make me feel sorry I ate it afterwards.

When I started to experiment with this brownie recipe, I wanted to add nuts into the batter because I love nuts in everything! But I needed to find out first if the brownie would be moist, and if the texture would be pleasing.

You can serve these brownies with a scoop of frozen yogurt or dairy-free ice cream!

MAKES 2 DOZEN

INGREDIENTS FOR THE CHOCOLATE SAUCE

4 ounces bittersweet chocolate, finely chopped
1 cup coconut oil, melted
1 tablespoon vanilla extract

INSTRUCTIONS

1. In a double boiler, melt the chocolate, 1 cup coconut oil, and 1 tablespoon of vanilla. Use a wooden spoon to mix until the chocolate has melted completely. Remove from the heat; cool for 20 minutes.

2. Pour into a food grade plastic needle-nose bottle (available online). Pour any remaining sauce into a glass container and store in refrigerator.

INGREDIENTS FOR THE BROWNIES

Organic coconut cooking spray

1 cup garbanzo-fava bean flour

¼ cup potato starch

2 tablespoons arrowroot

½ cup unsweetened organic cocoa powder

1 cup monk fruit sugar

¼ teaspoon baking soda

2 teaspoons baking powder

¼ teaspoon xanthan gum

1 teaspoon kosher salt

1 cup coconut oil, melted

½ cup applesauce

2½ tablespoons vanilla extract, divided

2 shots espresso or ½ cup strong brewed coffee

1¼ cups organic chocolate chips

½ cup chopped walnuts

Edible flowers, for garnish (available online, optional)

INSTRUCTIONS

1. Preheat the oven to 325F°.

2. Generously spray a 9 × 9-inch baking pan. (I use a muffin tin shaped with 12 squares.) Spray the squares with the coconut oil.

3. In a medium bowl, mix the garbanzo-fava flour, potato starch, arrowroot, cocoa powder, monk fruit sugar, baking soda, baking powder, xanthan gum, and salt.

4. In a bowl, pour the remaining cup of coconut oil, applesauce, 2½ tablespoons of vanilla, and coffee, and mix together. Add to the flour mixtures; stir until the batter is smooth. Using a rubber spatula, gently fold in the chocolate chips and walnuts.

5. Pour the batter into the baking pan or use a tablespoon to scoop the batter into each muffin cup ¾ full. Bake on the center rack for 8 minutes.

6. Remove the brownies from the oven and let stand in the pans for 10 minutes to cool. Cut the brownies into squares. If you're using muffin tins, remove the brownies and place on a baking sheet.

7. Drizzle chocolate sauce over the brownies and arrange on a serving plate.

Tip: Xanthan gum is available at health food stores and some supermarkets.

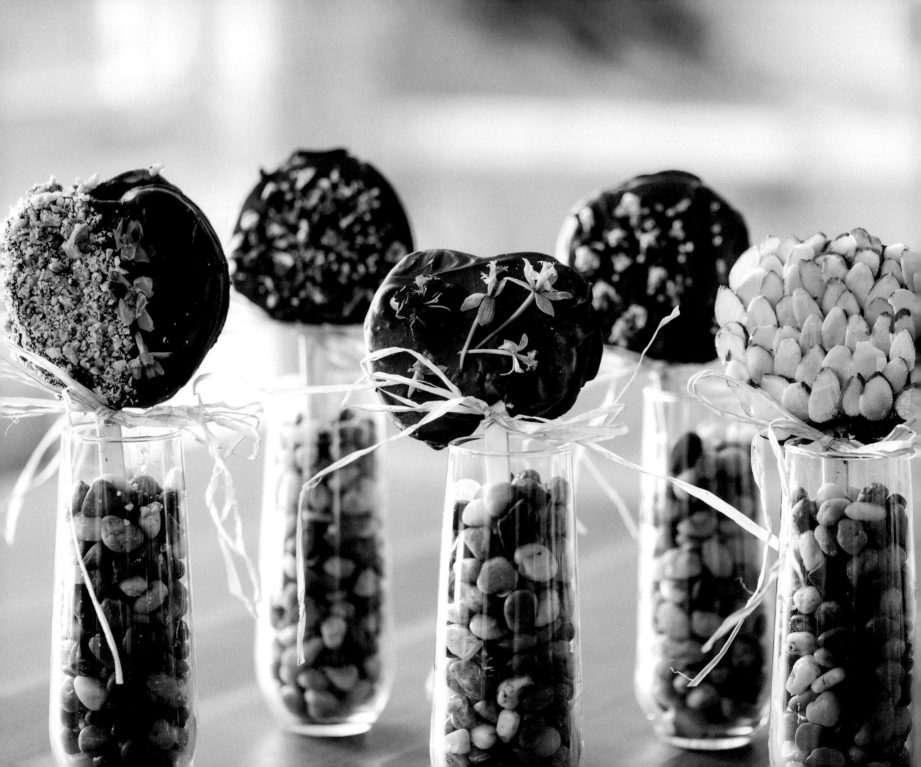

Chocolate Turtle Apple Slices

What is better than a cold slice of apple dipped in chocolate? These are easy to make and so much fun to do. Alex, Ari, and I had so much fun decorating our apples. They also make great table decorations. These can be frozen and enjoyed right out of the freezer!

MAKES 10 TO 12 SLICES

INGREDIENTS

4 cups Ghirardelli dark chocolate chips

1 tablespoon coconut oil

2 large unpeeled green apples, sliced into ¾-inch pieces

12 popsicle sticks

1 cup store-bought caramel sauce, poured into a plastic needle nose bottle

1½ cups chopped pecans or walnuts

INSTRUCTIONS

1. Line a cookie sheet with parchment paper.

2. In a double boiler, combine the chocolate chips and coconut oil. Melt the chocolate until it's smooth. Use a wooden spoon to mix.

3. With a paring knife make a small slit in the bottom of each apple slice and insert a popsicle stick.

4. Dip the apple slices into the melted chocolate and place on the parchment-lined cookie sheet. Drizzle a tiny bit of the caramel sauce over the apple slices and sprinkle with nuts. Refrigerate 1 hour to set the chocolate.

5. You can have fun decorating your apple slices. I've included some decorating examples in the photograph.

6. The apples should be eaten the same day. If you don't eat them first day (which is impossible, of course!), cover with wrap and store them in the refrigerator. They will keep for 2 days.

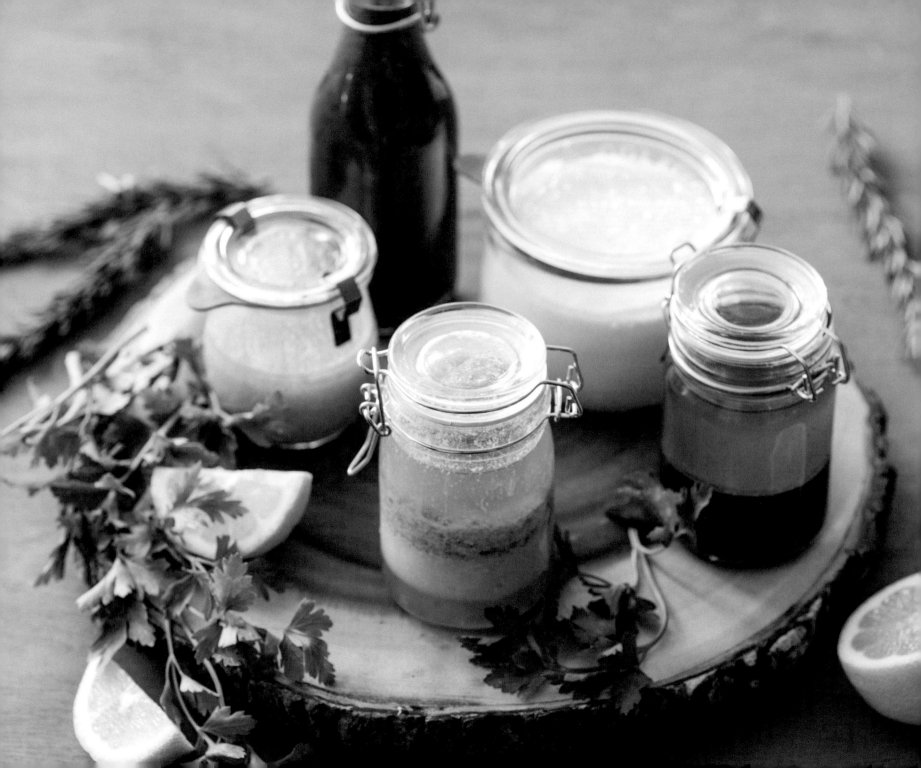

CHAPTER 10

Vinaigrettes
& Salad Dressings

Creamy Shallot Vinaigrette

This is a lovely dressing for salads that feature tender produce such as butter lettuce, baby greens, arugula, and tomatoes. It also makes a great marinade for chicken, turkey, and fish. This dressing will keep up to 4 days in the refrigerator.

MAKES 1 CUP

INGREDIENTS

1 heaping tablespoon Dijon mustard
¾ cup extra-virgin olive oil
1 tablespoon minced shallots
3 tablespoons Champagne vinegar
2 tablespoons fresh lemon juice
1 teaspoon kosher salt

INSTRUCTIONS

In a blender, combine the Dijon mustard and olive oil; blend 30 seconds to emulsify. Pour into a bowl and add the shallots, Champagne vinegar, lemon juice, and salt. Whisk until smooth and creamy.

Avocado Dressing

MAKES 1 CUP

INGREDIENTS

1 medium avocado, peeled, pitted, and cut into chunks

2 tablespoons cashew cream or cashew milk

½ cup canned unsweetened coconut milk

2 tablespoons fresh lime juice

½ of a small clove of garlic, smashed

1 tablespoon fresh dill

1 tablespoon chives, finely chopped

½ teaspoon kosher salt

⅛ teaspoon cayenne pepper

INSTRUCTIONS

Process the avocado, cashew cream or milk, coconut milk, lime juice, and garlic in a blender for 30 seconds. Transfer to a small bowl and stir in the dill, chives, salt, and cayenne pepper.

Raspberry Vinaigrette

MAKES ¾ CUP

INGREDIENTS

½ cup extra-virgin olive oil

2 tablespoons walnut oil

2 teaspoons finely chopped shallots

2 tablespoons rice wine vinegar

1 tablespoon malt vinegar

4 tablespoons raspberry vinegar

½ teaspoon kosher salt

⅛ teaspoon cracked black pepper

INSTRUCTIONS

In a glass bowl, whisk the olive oil, walnut oil, shallots, rice wine vinegar, malt vinegar, raspberry vinegar, salt, and pepper. Store in an airtight glass container in the refrigerator. The vinaigrette will keep up to 3 days.

Asian Citrus Vinaigrette

Use as a dressing over salads, as a marinade for chicken or pork, or as a stir-fry sauce with a little cornstarch added to thicken the sauce.

MAKES 1¼ CUPS

INGREDIENTS

1 cup orange juice

1 tablespoon lime juice

2 tablespoons soy sauce

1 tablespoon honey

½ teaspoon Sriracha hot sauce

1 small garlic clove, peeled and smashed

1 tablespoon grated fresh ginger

½ teaspoon kosher salt

1 tablespoon sesame oil

3 tablespoons extra-virgin olive oil

INSTRUCTIONS

In a blender or food processor, blend the orange juice, lime juice, soy sauce, honey, Sriracha hot sauce, garlic, ginger, and salt. Slowly add the sesame and olive oils, with the blender running on medium until all of the oils have been added.

Blue Cheese Dressing

MAKES 1½ CUPS

INGREDIENTS

⅔ cup buttermilk

1 cup low-fat sour cream

2 tablespoons Champagne vinegar

2 tablespoons fresh lemon juice

6 ounces high quality blue cheese, crumbled

⅛ teaspoon cayenne pepper

1 teaspoon kosher salt

INSTRUCTIONS

1. Whisk the buttermilk and sour cream until smooth. Add the vinegar and lemon juice; whisk. Fold the blue cheese into the buttermilk mixture. Add the cayenne pepper and salt; mix gently.

2. Store in the refrigerator in an airtight glass container. This dressing will keep in the refrigerator for 3 days.

Balsamic Vinaigrette

MAKES 1¼ CUPS

INGREDIENTS

¾ cup extra-virgin olive oil

1 heaping tablespoon Dijon mustard

1 tablespoon finely chopped shallots

¼ cup aged balsamic vinegar

¼ cup red wine vinegar

2 tablespoons low-sodium soy sauce
or tamari (gluten-free soy sauce)

3 tablespoons rice wine vinegar

2 tablespoons apple cider vinegar

3 tablespoons fresh lemon juice

1 tablespoon maple syrup

1 teaspoon each kosher salt and cracked black pepper

1 garlic clove, peeled and smashed

INSTRUCTIONS

Place the olive oil, Dijon mustard, shallots, balsamic vinegar, red wine vinegar, soy sauce, rice wine vinegar, apple cider vinegar, lemon juice, maple syrup, salt, and pepper in a glass jar. Shake well. Add the garlic and cover tightly with lid. The vinaigrette will keep in the refrigerator for 3 days.

Caesar Dressing

MAKES 1 CUP

INGREDIENTS

3 anchovy fillets

1 garlic clove, peeled

½ cup extra-virgin olive oil

¼ cup Dijon mustard

½ cup fresh lemon juice

2 tablespoons Worcestershire sauce

¼ teaspoon each kosher salt and cracked black pepper

INSTRUCTIONS

Place the anchovies, garlic, olive oil, Dijon mustard, lemon juice, Worcestershire sauce, salt, and pepper in a blender. Blend for 30 seconds. It will be perfectly mixed—smooth, and creamy! Enjoy.

Champagne Vinaigrette

MAKES ¾ CUP

INGREDIENTS

¼ cup Champagne vinegar
1 tablespoon Dijon mustard
½ teaspoon kosher salt
¼ teaspoon ground black pepper
1 tablespoon organic honey
½ cup extra-virgin olive oil

INSTRUCTIONS

In a small bowl, whisk the Champagne vinegar, Dijon mustard, salt, pepper, and honey. While continuing to whisk, slowly add the olive oil until the vinaigrette is emulsified.

Balsamic Glaze

MAKES ⅓ CUP

INGREDIENTS

1 bottle (16.9-ounce) balsamic vinegar

INSTRUCTIONS

Pour the entire bottle of balsamic vinegar into a small saucepan and bring to a boil over high heat. Lower the heat to medium-high and continue to boil until the vinegar starts to thicken and forms a syrup-like consistency, about 14 to 20 minutes. Be careful not to let it thicken too much, or you will end up with a thick black goop.

Tip: To test, use a wooden spoon: If the syrup coats the back of the spoon it is ready to be removed from the heat. Let it cool to room temperature before you store it. I use a needle-nose plastic bottle to store the glaze after it has cooled. It will last up to a month in the refrigerator.

Lemon Vinaigrette

SERVES 6

INGREDIENTS

½ cup extra-virgin olive oil

¼ cup fresh lemon juice

⅓ cup fresh orange juice

½ teaspoon each kosher salt and cracked black pepper

¼ teaspoon ground cumin

INSTRUCTIONS

Combine the olive oil, lemon juice, orange juice, salt, pepper, and cumin in a jar with a tightly fitting lid. Shake vigorously to thoroughly mix.

Raw Apple Cider Vinaigrette

This dressing is great on salads with fruit or peppery greens like watercress and arugula. Apple cider vinegar has many health benefits including lowering glucose levels, and helping with gas, bloating, and heartburn. It has an alkalizing effect, which helps with gut health.

MAKES 1 CUP

INGREDIENTS

½ cup extra-virgin olive oil

1 tablespoon Dijon mustard

¾ cup raw apple cider vinegar

2 tablespoons fresh lemon juice

2 tablespoons raw honey

½ teaspoon kosher salt

I garlic clove, peeled and smashed

INSTRUCTIONS

Combine the olive oil, Dijon mustard, apple cider vinegar, lemon juice, honey, and salt in a glass Mason jar. Cover tightly with the lid and shake until the honey has dissolved. Add the garlic; seal tightly. Store in the refrigerator for up to 4 days.

Tip: When you shop for apple cider vinegar, make sure the label says, "With the Mother." These are raw enzymes and gut-friendly bacteria that are thought to promote healing. My go-to brand is Bragg's.

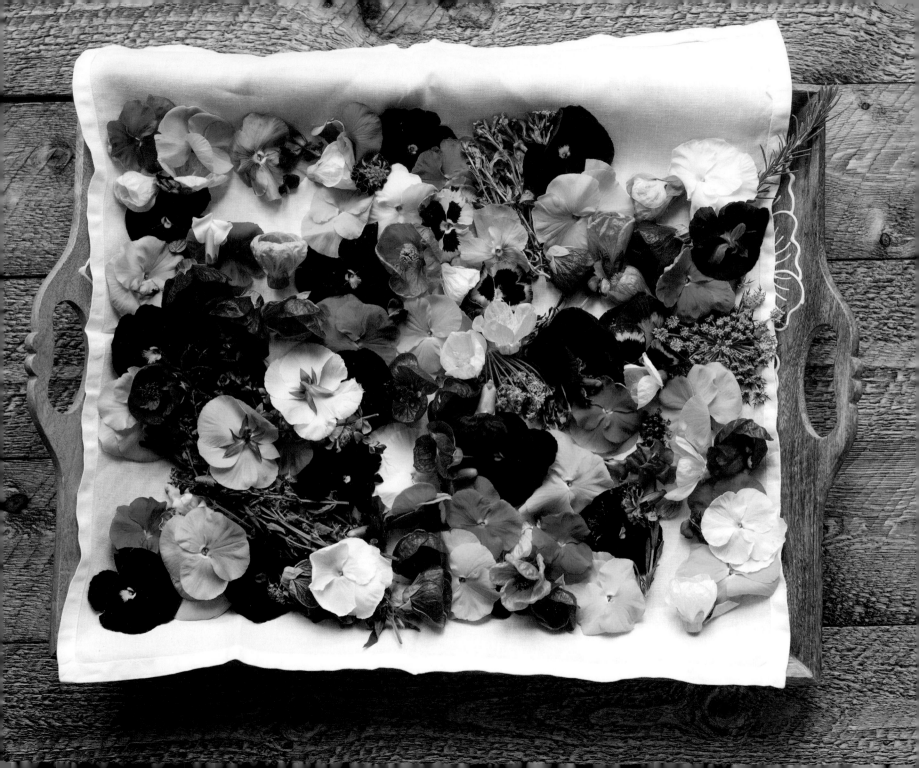

CHAPTER 11

Salsas, Sauces & Garnishes

Sriracha Mayo

MAKES ½ CUP

INGREDIENTS

½ cup regular or vegan mayonnaise
3 tablespoons lemon juice
2 tablespoons Sriracha hot sauce

INSTRUCTIONS

In a small bowl, combine the mayonnaise, lemon juice, and Sriracha hot sauce. Mix well. Cover tightly and refrigerate to chill for 30 minutes.

Tomato Salsa

MAKES ABOUT 4 CUPS

INGREDIENTS

3 cups (around 12 to 14) peeled, seeded,
   and diced Roma tomatoes
½ cup diced red onion
¼ cup loosely packed cilantro, finely chopped
2 scallions, white and light green part, finely chopped
2 tablespoons fresh lime juice
1 teaspoon kosher salt
1 jalapeño, finely diced, with seeds
2 tablespoons extra-virgin olive oil

INSTRUCTIONS

1. Place the tomatoes, onion, cilantro, scallions, lime juice, salt, jalapeño, and olive oil in a glass bowl. Mix well.

2. Refrigerate, covered, in an airtight glass container for at least 3 to 4 hours. The salsa can be made the day before and will last 3 to 4 days in the refrigerator in an airtight container.

Salsa Verde

MAKES ABOUT 2 CUPS

INGREDIENTS

1 bunch Italian (flat leaf) parsley, finely chopped
1 shallot, minced
¼ cup red wine vinegar
1 cup plus 4 tablespoons extra-virgin olive oil
½ teaspoon each kosher salt and cracked black pepper
2 anchovies
¼ teaspoon crushed red pepper
2 teaspoons honey
2 teaspoons fresh mint, finely chopped
1 tablespoon capers, rinsed and drained
2 teaspoons lemon zest

INSTRUCTIONS

In a glass bowl, add the parsley, shallot, vinegar, olive oil, salt, pepper, anchovies, crushed red pepper, honey, mint, capers, and lemon zest. Mix together and store in a glass container with a lid. Store in the refrigerator until ready to use. Salsa will keep for 3 days.

Cucumber-Yogurt Sauce

MAKES ABOUT 2½ CUPS

INGREDIENTS

1 cucumber, peeled, seeded, and chopped
    into small pieces
2 cups plain whole-milk Greek yogurt
3 tablespoons extra-virgin olive oil
2 tablespoons fresh lemon juice
1 tablespoon fresh mint, finely chopped
1 tablespoon fresh dill
1 small garlic clove, minced
½ teaspoon kosher salt
½ teaspoon ground black pepper

INSTRUCTIONS

1. Place the cucumber into a bowl and add the yogurt, olive oil, lemon juice, mint, dill, garlic, salt, and pepper. Mix well. Cover and refrigerate 30 minutes before serving.

2. Cucumber-Yogurt Sauce will last for 3 days in the refrigerator in an airtight container.

Arugula Pesto

MAKES 1 CUP

INGREDIENTS

4 cups arugula, washed and dried well
1 small garlic clove, peeled
1 cup extra-virgin olive oil
½ cup grated Parmesan cheese
½ teaspoon kosher salt
1 tablespoon lemon zest

INSTRUCTIONS

1. In a blender or food processor, add the arugula and garlic; process 15 seconds. Stop the blender or food processor and add the olive oil, Parmesan cheese, and salt. Pulse-chop to incorporate the ingredients. Don't over blend—you don't want a thick paste.

2. Add the lemon zest and use a spoon to mix it through. Pour into a Mason jar and cover tightly.

Tip: Try to eat pesto the day you make it; the flavors will be bright and super fresh. Arugula Pesto will last up to 2 days in the refrigerator. But don't leave *any* pesto in the refrigerator for more than 2 days. Garlic is a living organism and will grow mold after a few days, and so will the cheese.

My Homemade Smokin' Barbecue Sauce

MAKES 1¼ QUARTS

INGREDIENTS

1 (28-ounce) can tomato purée
1 cup white wine vinegar
½ cup honey
¼ cup unsulphured organic molasses
4 tablespoons paprika
1 tablespoon onion powder
1 tablespoon garlic powder
1 tablespoon ground cumin
1 tablespoon kosher salt
1 tablespoon ground black pepper

INSTRUCTIONS

1. In a saucepan, whisk the tomato purée, vinegar, honey, molasses, paprika, onion powder, garlic powder, cumin, salt, and pepper.

2. On high heat, bring the mixture to a boil. Reduce the heat to low; simmer 30 minutes. Remove from heat and allow the sauce to cool to room temperature.

3. Use immediately or refrigerate until ready to use.

Tip: Smokin' Barbecue Sauce will keep in the refrigerator in an airtight glass container for up to a week.

Pickled Red Onion

MAKES ABOUT 2 CUPS

INGREDIENTS

1 tablespoon apple cider vinegar
1 tablespoon monk fruit sweetener
1½ teaspoon kosher salt
1 cup water
1 red onion, thinly sliced

INSTRUCTIONS

1. Whisk the vinegar, monk fruit, and salt with 1 cup water in a small glass bowl until the salt dissolves.

2. Place the onions in a Mason jar or other lidded glass jar. Pour the vinegar mixture over them and cover tightly with the lid. Let it sit at room temperature for at least an hour. Store in the refrigerator.

Roasted Pumpkin Seeds

Nuts and seeds, including pumpkin seeds, are rich in certain plant-based chemicals called phytosterols that have been shown in studies to reduce LDL or "bad cholesterol." A diet rich in phytosterols is a great way to reduce your risk of heart disease. And now, researchers believe that phytosterols also play a role in prevention of Alzheimer's disease as well. This is great news, since I love roasted pumpkin seeds. I put them on everything— in my yogurt, salads, soups, and just plain as a snack.

MAKES ABOUT 2 CUPS

INGREDIENTS

1 teaspoon salt, divided

2 cups pumpkin seeds

1 tablespoon extra-virgin olive oil

½ teaspoon garlic powder

½ teaspoon onion powder

¼ teaspoon cayenne pepper

½ teaspoon black pepper

½ teaspoon chili powder

½ teaspoon ground cumin

INSTRUCTIONS

1. Preheat the oven to 350F°.

2. Fill a small saucepan with water and add ½ teaspoon kosher salt. Bring the water to a boil, add the pumpkin seeds, and let boil for 10 to 12 minutes. Drain.

3. Pour the seeds onto paper towels and pat dry. Place into a bowl, add the olive oil, and toss to coat the seeds evenly.

4. In a small bowl, whisk the garlic powder, onion powder, ½ teaspoon salt, cayenne pepper, pepper, chili powder, and cumin. Add the pumpkin seeds. Toss, making sure to coat the seeds.

5. Spread the seeds evenly on a baking sheet and bake 15 to 20 minutes, checking every 10 minutes to make sure they are not burning. Shake the baking sheet halfway through roasting. Remove from the oven and cool.

Cook's Note: If you are using a fresh pumpkin, scrape out the seeds. Make sure to remove any pumpkin rind and slimy threads. Soak in a bowl of cool water for 1 hour to clean the seeds. Drain before using.

Toasted Walnuts

Walnuts pick up an earthy, rich flavor if they are toasted first.

MAKES 4 CUPS

INGREDIENTS

4 cups of chopped walnuts

INSTRUCTIONS

1. Place into a cold, dry frying pan and turn the heat to medium.

2. Shake the pan back and forth every few moments until the walnuts start to release their oils and turn a beautiful golden rich brown, 3 to 4 minutes.

Tip: Be careful not to burn the walnuts or they will taste bitter. If that happens, you need to toss them and start over. Store in an airtight container.

Toasted Coconut

MAKES 2 CUPS

INGREDIENTS

2 cups shredded coconut

INSTRUCTIONS

1. Preheat the oven to 350F°. Place 2 cups shredded coconut on a baking sheet and spread evenly.

2. Bake until the coconut starts to toast, 5 to 10 minutes. Watch carefully; once it starts to toast, it will brown quickly.

3. Remove and set aside in separate small bowl.

Croutons

MAKES 4 CUPS

INGREDIENTS

4 cups cubed sourdough bread

2 tablespoons extra-virgin olive oil

INSTRUCTIONS

1. Preheat the oven to 350F°. Place the sourdough bread into a medium-sized bowl. Drizzle it with the olive oil and use your hands to mix.

2. Bake in a preheated oven on a baking sheet for 10 to 15 minutes or until the cubes are crunchy and turn a golden color.

3. Let cool. Store in an airtight container. Croutons will keep for 3 weeks.

Ghee (Clarified Butter)

MAKES ABOUT 5 OUNCES

INGREDIENTS

8 ounces (1 stick) unsalted butter

INSTRUCTIONS

1. In a small saucepan over low heat, melt, allowing the butter to melt undisturbed. When the butter has melted, carefully remove the foam that has formed on top with a spoon.

2. Pour the clear yellow liquid into a glass Mason jar. Be careful not to let the solids (white congealed matter) at the bottom get into the jar with the clarified butter. The solids will burn and turn brown at high temperatures, so discard the them too.

3. Cover tightly and store in the refrigerator.

Spicy Mango Salsa

MAKES ABOUT 3 CUPS

INGREDIENTS

1 ripe mango (1 cup) peeled, pitted, and chopped into small pieces

1 cucumber, peeled, seeded, and diced

1 tablespoon finely diced jalapeño, seeds removed, optional

¼ cup red bell pepper, seeded and diced

¼ teaspoon crushed red pepper

1 scallion trimmed, cut into thin rings

2 tablespoons extra-virgin olive oil

2 tablespoons fresh lime juice

½ teaspoon kosher salt

2 teaspoons cilantro, finely chopped

6 mint leaves, finely chopped

INSTRUCTIONS

Place the mango, cucumber, jalapeño, bell pepper, crushed red pepper, scallion, olive oil, lime juice, salt, cilantro, and mint in a glass bowl or Mason jar. Mix thoroughly. Cover tightly and refrigerate. This salsa will last up to 3 days.

Ricotta Cheese

INGREDIENTS

2 quarts whole milk

1 cup heavy cream

½ teaspoon kosher salt

2 tablespoons fresh lemon juice

INSTRUCTIONS

1. Line a mesh strainer with a layer of cheesecloth and place it over a large bowl.

2. In a heavy medium-sized saucepan over medium-high heat, slowly bring the milk, cream, and salt to a rolling boil, stirring occasionally so it doesn't scorch.

3. Add the lemon juice. Reduce the heat to low and simmer, stirring constantly, until the mixture curdles, about 1 to 2 minutes.

4. Pour the mixture into the lined strainer and drain for 1 hour. Discard the liquid that collects in the bottom of the bowl along with the cheesecloth.

5. Cover the cheese tightly with plastic wrap. Chill thoroughly. It will keep for 2 days in the refrigerator.

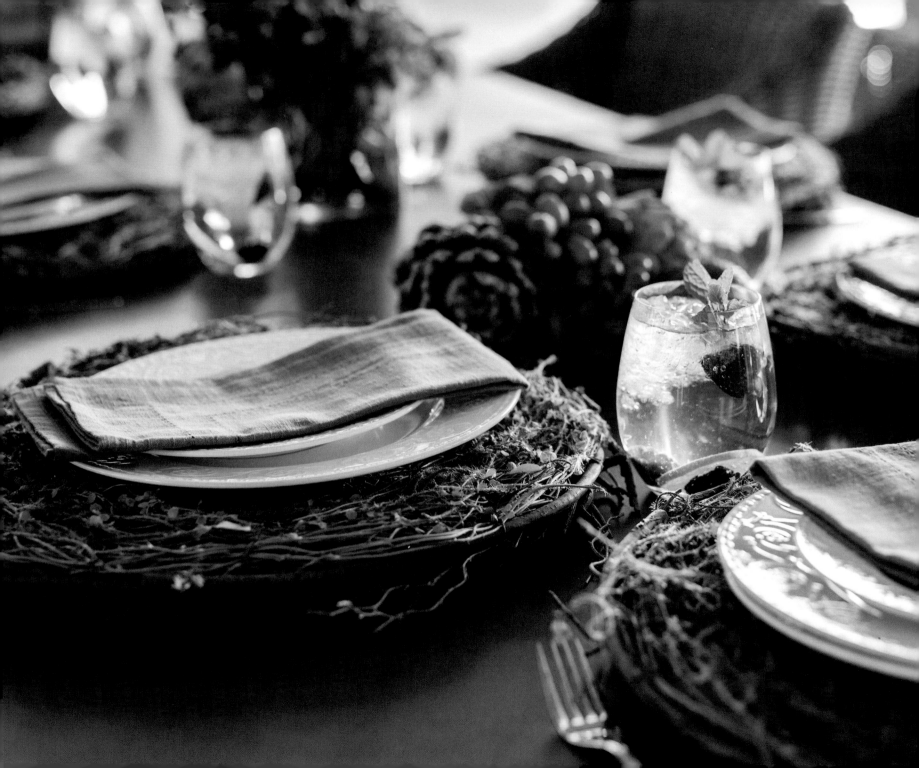

Acknowledgments

Thank you to God who guides my every step of this magnificent journey that is my life. I may have not liked some of the struggles, trials, and things I did not understand at the time, but I became the woman I always wanted to be. I am blessed and filled with gratitude.

Tony, my husband, who is the best part of me, of us, of our family. Completing this book was an obsession of mine, and Tony understood how important this project was to me. When I got sick with cancer and had to put everything on hold for a year, he never left my side and took control without taking mine away. He circled the wagons and worked on his own projects while never taking his eyes off me. He kept us all together, strong, united, sane, and made us feel safe. A greater love in my life I have never known.

Alexandra and Arianna Thomopoulos, I can't even begin to express the pure joy it was for me to have my daughters involved in this book. They are both extremely busy, in-demand working women who gave up many weekends and weekdays to help me with the beautiful photos for this book. We shot over 120 fully prepped and styled photographs. We kitchen tested each recipe, laughed, ate, gained weight, and created more beautiful memories! Thank you, my loves! I'm only sorry my daughter, Kathryn, who lives in Texas, was not here to be with me during the shoot for this book. Next one,

Ka Ka, for sure! Your boundless energy and positivity was missed!

Kathryn, Anne, Mark, Denis, Alexandra, Arianna, Claire, Kevin, Kasey, Sera, Jason, Neil, my reason for living.

Maria Shriver, my dear friend, I stare at those words, "my friend." I can't believe that this extraordinary woman is part of my life. Our families have been through a lot over our 30 years of friendship, none more than hers. She is my example of grace under fire, my mentor, my role model. Fiercely loyal, loving, supportive, kind, funny, and in your face big time if she needs to be. She picked me up off the floor at one of the lowest points in my life. Her phone call to me at that time changed everything. She acknowledged my pain, offered comforting words, and was angry for me. "Don't worry, you'll be fine. Come work with me on my Women's Alzheimer's Movement. Join me, let's figure out how we can use what you are doing with the new cookbook you are working on and use it to help people. Come do a Facebook Live with me and we can share a recipe from the book." The Facebook Live was a huge success right out of the box. We talked about food and health and the effects of food on the body and brain. The response was overwhelming. It changed my life and purpose. That's how *Food for Thought* came to be. My friend opened up this new path in my life. She stands by me with support and love, as always, all these many years. Thank you, Maria. Onward...

Jan Miller, one of my closest and most cherished friends. I met Jan over 30 years ago when she became my literary agent, and she has since championed 6 books for me. I don't know anyone like Jan Miller. We share an unusual connection that, frankly, neither of us quite understands. We are connected on a level that transcends reason. We blend into each other like a liquid that is warm, comforting, and homogenized. We finish each other sentences, laugh until we are exhausted and in a ball on the floor, and when we hug we are one. I simply love you, Jan, beyond reason and I cannot adequately describe how blessed I am that you are in my life. I am a better woman, wife, mother, and friend because of your example. You live life large and you're a supernova bringing light and love across the lives of everyone whose path you cross.

My sister, Diana, and brother, Gino, for their love, support, and prayers. My connection to everything in my life that is meaningful,

God, love of family, for being there for one another, and our many, many children and grandchildren we share. Mom and Dad would have been so proud, but I think they know.

Marina Ponce, always by my side in our home. I am grateful beyond words that for over 30 years this wonderful God-sent woman has helped me keep my life and our home running smoothly. This is the third cookbook that she has helped me with and they all have been challenging, in a good way. The craziness in the kitchen for weeks testing over 200 recipes was beyond reason. Then the actual shooting of the photographs. She kept us all on track, calm and organized. Marina, we love, cherish, and appreciate you. Thank you for everything you do for me and our family.

Katina Beach, my soulmate sister, for all of the support and unconditional love you give me and my family every single day. Thank you for the use of your beautiful home for some of the beautiful photography in this book. Thanks for being my taste tester and kitchen tester for most of the recipes. Thanks for your input and honesty. Thanks for making me laugh, praying for me, and giving me words of encouragement to put one foot in front of the other and not complain.

Maria Lerios, my other soulmate sister who is actually the *real* sister of Katina Beach. Maria is a tiny powerhouse of a woman, and a cornerstone of strength, dignity, and loyalty mixed in with a bit of rebellion, which I just love about you. You are a fiercely loyal friend and protector of those you love. Thanks for your continued love and support during the struggles of continuing this book while I was ill. You helped me stay focused, prayed for me, made me laugh, and helped champion me to the finish line. I love when the three of us are out together and I stand a foot taller than the two of you and people ask if we are sisters. I am the first to shout out proudly, "Yes, I'm the tall one!" I love you and your family beyond words and look forward to every family occasion we share.

Suzy Graham, a fairly new friend who God put in my path these past few years. Her kindness, support, and weekly inspiration helped me during my illness and brought me great comfort and healing. I met her one day when I wandered into her home furnishing and accessories boutique. We became instant "best friends." I used many of the beautiful accessories from her store, Bricks and Beams, that she so graciously loaned to me to style the exceptional photographs in this book. Thank you, sweet Suzy. I thank God for bringing you into my life.

Todd and Diane, you are two of the sweetest, kindest, generous, most exceptional people with whom I have ever had the pleasure to know and work with. We ended up with a friendship that I cherish. I met Diane and Todd when they photographed my last cookbook *Big Bowl of Love*. The experience was life changing for me as they taught me everything I know about food styling, which has become my passion. Shooting over 120 photos is no small feat, but their patience, love, and passion for what they do shows in every photo. We had fun, no stress, and pure joy, and we ate well. I am so proud of this book, but the images are what makes this cookbook, in my opinion, exceptional.

Thank you, Anthony Ziccardi, Publisher of Post Hill Press, for believing in my vision for this book. I can't thank you enough for your support. Thank you for helping me get the word out about food and health and the connection between diet and overall body health, something I am truly passionate about. I want you to know that the "Sandwich" chapter was created for you after you told me how much you love sandwiches, and asked if there would be any in the book. Now you have a whole chapter to choose from!

Maddie Sturgeon, what a pure pleasure it has been working with you. You are an amazing person to work with, and you kept me calm, focused, and excited throughout the whole process. I sincerely hope we will have another chance to do this again! Many thanks Maddie! Big hugs!

I saved my Annie Gilbar for last and have a whole page just for her. My morning starts at the crack of dawn with my friend and heart light Annie. It comes in the form of a text that wakes me with that annoying trumpet sound. (I need to change that.) "How are you feeling today, pumpkin?" which is followed 10 minutes later with a phone call. Annie is the first voice I hear in the morning and the last one I hear before I go to sleep. She checks in with me at least 2 more times during the day and we discuss the news of the day, family, the cookbook, her business, my business. She is on top of everything and my go-to person for everything I do in my life. Annie is my connection to reason, to thoughtfulness, to giving of oneself without asking for anything in return. She just does stuff from the goodness of her huge heart. Whenever there is a crisis with me, my family, or the friends she loves, she is *the first person* to be there unconditionally. When I told her I had multiple myeloma, cancer of the plasma cells, before I could digest the news, she wrote a list for me with names of the best doctors all over the country, the best hospitals, research for me to read, and a phone call she just happened to arrange for me with Tom Brokaw, who has the same cancer. "Here's his number, call him, he's waiting to talk to you." That phone call changed everything and put me on the path to wellness. You are a blessing in my life. My heart is full. I love you Fanny!

References

"7 Benefits of Eating Walnuts | Walnut's Nutrition." 2018. Mercola.com. Accessed July 18. https://articles.mercola.com/sites/articles/archive/2014/05/19/7-walnuts-benefits.aspx.

"7 Health Benefits of Cantaloupe." 2017. Eat This! June 1. http://www.healthdiaries.com/eatthis/7-health-benefits-of-cantaloupe.html.

"7 Health Benefits of Cashews." 2017. Eat This! January 4. http://www.healthdiaries.com/eat-this/7-health-benefits-of-cashews.html.

"7 Health Benefits of Walnut Oil." 2015. Eat This! August 7. http://www.healthdiaries.com/eatthis/7-health-benefits-of-walnut-oil.html.

"8 Health Benefits of Hazelnuts." 2015. Eat This! August 5. http://www.healthdiaries.com/eatthis/8-health-benefits-of-hazelnuts.html.

"10 Amazing Benefits of Artichokes." 2018. Organic Facts. Organic Facts. May 15. https://www.organicfacts.net/health-benefits/other/health-benefits-of-artichokes.html.

"10 Impressive Benefits of Carrots." 2018. Organic Facts. Organic Facts. July 11. https://www.organicfacts.net/health-benefits/vegetable/carrots.html.

"13 Amazing Benefits of Apple." 2018. Organic Facts. Organic Facts. July 11. https://www.organicfacts.net/health-benefits/fruit/health-benefits-of-apple.html.

"15 Impressive Fennel Benefits." 2018. Organic Facts. Organic Facts. July 17. https://www.organicfacts.net/health-benefits/herbs-and-spices/health-benefits-of-fennel.html.

"16 Health Benefits of Rosemary." 2017. Eat This! June 1. http://www.healthdiaries.com/eatthis/16-health-benefits-of-rosemary.html.

"The American Heart Association's Diet and Lifestyle Recommendations." 2018. How Cigarettes Damage Your Body. Accessed July 18. http://www.heart.org/HEARTORG/HealthyLiving/HealthyEating/Nutrition/The-American-Heart-Associations-Diet-and-Lifestyle-Recommendations_UCM_305855_Article.jsp#.W0-jui_MzVp.

Barrett, Mike. 2014. "12 Health Benefits of Sesame Seeds and Sesame Oil." Natural Society. May 21. http://naturalsociety.com/12-health-benefits-of-sesame-seeds-sesame-oil/.

"Basil." 2018. Cabbage. Accessed July 19. http://www.whfoods.com/genpage.php?tname=foodspice&dbid=85.

"The Benefits of Coconut Oil." 2010. HowStuffWorks. HowStuffWorks. June 29. http://health.howstuffworks.com/wellness/food-nutrition/facts/benefits-of-coconut-oil.htm.

"Benefits of Eating Stone Fruits, Stone Fruits Recipes." 2016. Bel Marra Health - Breaking Health News and Health Information. Bel Marra Health. April 13. https://www.belmarrahealth.com/health-benefits-and-nutritional-facts-of-stone-fruits/.

"The Best Nuts for Your Heart." 2016. Mayo Clinic. Mayo Foundation for Medical Education and Research. September 15. https://www.mayoclinic.org/diseases-conditions/heart-disease/in-depth/nuts/art-20046635.

"Blueberries Reduce Risk of Parkinson's, Boost Brain Function Finds New Study." 2014. Plants for Human Health Institute. April 7. http://plantsforhumanhealth.ncsu.edu/2014/04/07/

blueberries-reduce-risk-of-parkinsons-boost-brain-function-finds-new-study/.

Boldt, Ethan. 2017. "Monk Fruit: Nature's Best Sweetener?" Dr. Axe. June 15. https://draxe.com/monk-fruit/.

Boldt, Ethan. 2017. "Health Benefits of Kale Kale Nutrition & Kale Recipes." Dr. Axe. July 5. https://draxe.com/health-benefits-of-kale/.

Borreli, Lizette. 2017. "7 Beets Benefits For Your Health, From Losing Weight To Better Sex." Medical Daily. July 24. https://www.medicaldaily.com/7-beets-benefits-your-health-losing-weight-better-sex-420462.

Brewer, Sarah. 2017. "Dr. Sarah Brewer Explains Benefits of Curry for Pain Relief." Daily Mail Online. Associated Newspapers. September 4. http://www.dailymail.co.uk/health/article-4834186/Can-curry-spice-really-help-banish-aches-pains.html.

Busch, Sandi. 2018. "What Are the Health Benefits of Anchovies." Healthy Eating | SF Gate. June 11. https://healthyeating.sfgate.com/health-benefits-anchovies-2748.html.

"Cantaloupe (Melon) Nutrition Facts and Health Benefits." 2018. Nutrition And You.com. Accessed July 18. http://www.nutrition-and-you.com/cantaloupe.html.

"CDC: U.S. Deaths from Heart Disease, Cancer on the Rise." 2016. News on Heart.org. August 24. https://news.heart.org/cdc-u-s-deaths-from-heart-disease-cancer-on-the-rise/.

Chan, Mae. 2014. "17 Reasons Why You Need a Mango Every Day." Health Impact News. February 19. http://healthimpactnews.com/2013/17-reasons-why-you-need-a-mango-every-day/.

"Cooking with Stainless Steel | Paleo Leap." 2015. Paleo Leap | Paleo Diet Recipes & Tips. September 27. https://paleoleap.com/cooking-stainless-steel/.

Corleone, Jill. 2017. "Nutritional Facts of Black Beans." LIVESTRONG.COM. Leaf Group. October 3. https://www.livestrong.com/article/238506-black-bean-nutritional-facts/.

Coyle, Daisy. 2017. "Is Nonstick Cookware Like Teflon Safe to Use?" Healthline. Healthline Media. July 13. https://www.healthline.com/nutrition/nonstick-cookware-safety.

Daniells, Stephen. 2013. "'Important' Study: Vitamin K Shows Benefits for Memory." Nutraingredients-Usa.com. William Reed Business Media Ltd. September 24. http://www.nutraIngredients-usa.com/Research/Important-study-Vitamin-K-shows-benefits-for-memory.

Daniluk, Julie. 2016. "Four Health Benefits of Limes." Chatelaine. February 22. http://www.chatelaine.com/health/diet/five-health-benefits-of-limes-they-can-reverse-the-signs-of-aging/.

"Definition of Omega-3 Fatty Acids." 2018. MedicineNet. Accessed July 18. https://www.medicinenet.com/script/main/art.asp?articlekey=13977.

"Dr. Weil–Integrative Medicine, Healthy Lifestyles & Happiness." 2018. DrWeil.com. DrWeil.com. July 11. http://www.drweil.com/drw/u/WBL02202/Breast-Cancer-Protection-from-Peaches-Plums.html.

Edwards, Rebekah. 2017. "Cancer-Preventing, Heart-Healthy, Brain-Boosting Lycopene." Dr. Axe. Dr. Axe. June 15. https://draxe.com/lycopene/.

Elliott, Brianna. 2017. "7 Impressive Health Benefits of Yogurt." Healthline. Healthline Media. January 20. https://www.healthline.com/nutrition/7-benefits-of-yogurt.

Emling, Shelley. 2015. "This Snack May Protect Against Memory Loss." *The Huffington Post*. TheHuffingtonPost.com. January 22. http://www.huffingtonpost.com/2015/01/22/walnuts-boost-memory-study_n_6525316.html.

"Facts and Figures." 2018. Alzheimer's Association. Alzheimer's Association. Accessed July 18. https://www.alz.org/alzheimers-dementia/facts-figures.

Fifield, Kathleen. 2017. "New Study Connection Between Diet and Alzheimer's." AARP. July 17. https://www.aarp.org/health/brain-health/info-2017/foods-decrease-alzheimers-risk-fd.html.

"Fish and Omega-3 Fatty Acids." 2016. How Cigarettes Damage Your Body. October 16. http://www.heart.org/HEARTORG/HealthyLiving/HealthyEating/HealthyDietGoals/Fish-and-Omega-3-Fatty-Acids_UCM_303248_Article.jsp#.W0--Ri_MzVp.

Fontenot, Beth. 2012. "The Benefits of Berries to the Brain." *The Atlantic*. Atlantic Media Company. April 3. http://www.theatlantic.com/health/archive/2012/04/the-benefits-of-berries-to-the-brain/255262/.

Fox, Maggie. 2015. "A Better Treatment for Alzheimer's: Exercise." NBCNews.com. NBCUniversal News Group. July 23. http://www.nbcnews.com/health/aging/better-treatment-alzheimers-exercise-n397461.

"Free Radical." 2018. Merriam-Webster. Merriam-Webster. Accessed July 18. https://www.merriam-webster.com/dictionary/free radical.

"Garlic." 2016. National Center for Complementary and Integrative Health. U.S. Department of Health and Human Services. November 30. https://nccih.nih.gov/health/garlic/ataglance.htm.

Gelman, Lauren. 2018. "7 Tricks to Make a Healthy Smoothie | Reader's Digest." Reader's Digest. Reader's Digest. Accessed July 18. https://www.rd.com/health/diet-weight-loss/7-tricks-to-make-a-healthy-smoothie/.

Grant, Stacey. 2017. "What Are the Health Benefits of the Anthocyanins in Blueberries?" LIVESTRONG.COM. Leaf Group. October 3. https://www.livestrong.com/article/345698-what-are-the-health-benefits-of-the-anthocyanins-in-blueberries/.

"Grapeseed Oil Benefits, Uses, Side Effects, Facts and Information." 2018. Hemp Oil: Benefits, Nutrition, Side Effects and Facts. Accessed July 18. http://www.seedguides.info/grapeseed-oil/.

Group, Edward. 2015. "Why Is Refined Sugar So Bad for Your Health?" Dr. Group's Healthy Living Articles. Global Healing Center, Inc. June 8. http://www.globalhealingcenter.com/sugar-problem/refined-sugar-the-sweetest-poison-of-all.

Group, Edward. 2015. "15 Foods With Vitamin E." Dr. Group's Healthy Living Articles. Global Healing Center, Inc. November 25. http://www.globalhealingcenter.com/natural-health/vitamin-e-foods/.

Harvard Health Publishing. 2015. "Glycemic Index for 60 Foods - Harvard Health." Harvard Health Blog. February. https://www.health.harvard.edu/diseases-and-conditions/glycemic-index-and-glycemic-load-for-100-foods.

Harvard Health Publishing. 2016. "Cancer and Diet: What's the Connection? - Harvard Health." Harvard Health Blog. September. https://www.health.harvard.edu/cancer/cancer-and-diet-whats-the-connection.

HealWithFood.org. 2018. "Health Benefits of Cannellini Beans." Radish Sprouts: Health Benefits and Nutrition Facts. Accessed July 18. http://www.healwithfood.org/health-benefits/cannellini-beans.php.

"The Health Benefits of Halibut - Check Your Food." 2018. Ingredient - Acorns - Check Your Food. Accessed July 18. https://www.checkyourfood.com/Infographic/Item?seoTitle=the-health-benefits-of-halibut.

"Health Benefits of Matcha Tea." 2018. Matcha Source. Accessed July 18. https://matchasource.com/health-benefits-of-matcha-tea/.

"Health Benefits of Thyme, One of Nature's Top Antioxidant Foods." 2018. Antioxidants for Health and Longevity. Accessed July 19. http://www.antioxidants-for-health-and-longevity.com/health-benefits-of-thyme.html.

"Healthy Herbs Nutrition Facts and the Health Benefits of Herbs." 2018. Nutrition And You.com. Accessed July 18. https://www.nutrition-and-you.com/healthy-herbs.html.

Heather, James. 2010. "Seven Great Benefits of Walnut Oil." Medical Daily. August 4. http://www.medicaldaily.com/seven-great-benefits-walnut-oil-231697.

Heller, Samantha. 2011. "After-40 Nutrition: The Surprising Health Benefits of Beans." The Dr. Oz Show. The Dr. Oz Show. October 14. http://www.doctoroz.com/article/after-40-nutrition-surprising-health-benefits-beans.

Jessica. 2014. "5 Brazil Nuts Health Benefits." YouQueen. October 24. http://youqueen.com/life/health/5-brazil-nuts-health-benefits/.

Johnson, Jeremy J. 2011. Advances in Pediatrics. U.S. National Library of Medicine. June 1. http://www.ncbi.nlm.nih.gov/pmc/articles/PMC3070765/.

Joy, Traci. 2017. "Benefits of Phytosterols." LIVESTRONG. COM. Leaf Group. August 14. http://www.livestrong.com/article/26224-benefits-phytosterols/.

JungMar, Alyssa. 2018. "5 Health Benefits of Beans and 5 Surprising Risks | Reader's Digest." Reader's Digest. Reader's Digest. Accessed July 18. https://www.rd.com/health/conditions/health-benefits-of-beans/#slideshow=slide2.

Krishan, Shubhra. 2018. "8 Great Benefits of Onions | Care2 Healthy Living." Healthy Living. Accessed July 18. https://www.care2.com/greenliving/8-great-reasons-to-eat-more-onions.html.

Leech, Joe. 2017. "10 Delicious Herbs and Spices With Powerful Health Benefits." Gale - Enter Product Login. Healthline. June 4. https://bit.ly/2mwUf1p.

Lehman, Shereen, and Richard N. Fogoros. 2018. "Boost Your Heart Health With Olive Oil." Verywell Fit. May 18. http://nutrition.about.com/od/dietsformedicaldisorders/a/oliveoil.htm.

"Lemon/Limes." 2018. Cabbage. Accessed July 18. http://www.whfoods.com/genpage.php?tname=foodspice&dbid=27.

Levine, Beth. 2018. "Health Benefits of Curry." Grandparents.com. Accessed July 18. https://www.grandparents.com/health-and-wellbeing/health/health-benefits-turmeric.

Lewis, Alison. 2012. "Top 10 Health Benefits of Eating Kale." Mindbodygreen. mindbodygreen. April 2. https://www.mindbodygreen.com/0-4408/Top-10-Health-Benefits-of-Eating-Kale.html.

Link, Rachael. 2018. "12 Major Benefits of Ginger for Body & Brain." Dr. Axe. Dr. Axe. June 14. https://draxe.com/10-medicinal-ginger-health-benefits/.

Lipman, Frank. 2015. "Why You Should Eat Avocados Every Day (If You Aren't Already!)." Mindbodygreen. mindbodygreen. May 4. https://www.mindbodygreen.com/0-18602/why-you-should-eat-avocados-every-day-if-you-arent-already.html.

LoGiudice, Pina, Peter Bongiorno, and Siobhan Bleakney. 2016. "The Surprising Health Benefits of Coconut Oil." The Dr. Oz Show. The Dr. Oz Show. October 25. http://www.doctoroz.com/article/surprising-health-benefits-coconut-oil?page=1.

Magee, Elaine. 2018. "The Benefits of Yogurt." WebMD. WebMD. Accessed July 18. https://www.webmd.com/food-recipes/features/benefits-yogurt#1.

Makkieh, Khadejah. 2018. "Does Boiling Vegetables Deplete Their Nutritional Value?" Healthy Eating | SF Gate. June 11. https://healthyeating.sfgate.com/boiling-vegetables-deplete-nutritional-value-1438.html.

Mandal, Ananya. 2014. "What Are Tau Proteins?" News-Medical.net. News-Medical.net. October 21. http://www.news-medical.net/life-sciences/What-are-Tau-Proteins.aspx.

Marie, Joanne. 2018. "Grape Seed Oil Health Benefits." Healthy Eating | SF Gate. June 11. http://healthyeating.sfgate.com/grape-seed-oil-health-benefits-6827.html.

Martinac, Paula. 2018. "What Are the Benefits of Eating Pistachios." Healthy Eating | SF Gate. June 11. http://healthyeating.sfgate.com/benefits-eating-pistachios-1507.html.

McCoy, Kathleen. 2018. "Are Ghee Benefits Better Than Butter?" Dr. Axe. Dr. Axe. January 18. https://draxe.com/ghee-benefits/.

McDowell, Carly, and Marissa Laliberte. 2018. "Healthy Herbs That Can Boost Your Brain." Reader's Digest. Reader's Digest. Accessed July 19. http://www.rd.com/health/healthy-eating/4-best-herbs-for-the-brain/.

McIntosh, James. 2018. "Eggs: Health Benefits, Nutritional Facts, and Risks." Medical News Today. MediLexicon International. January 22. https://www.medicalnewstoday.com/articles/283659.php.

"More Information on Complementary and Alternative Medicine." 2018. American Cancer Society. Accessed July 18. http://www.cancer.org/treatment/treatmentsandsideeffects/complementaryandalternativemedicine/herbsvitaminsandminerals/molybdenum.

"MYTH: All Lettuce Is Good for You | Jillian Michaels." 2018. Jillianmichaels.com. Accessed July 18. https://www.jillianmichaels.com/blog/food-and-nutrition/myth-all-lettuce-good-you.

Nordqvist, Christian. 2017. "Olive Oil: Health Benefits, Nutritional Information." Medical News Today. MediLexicon International. December 11. http://www.medicalnewstoday.com/articles/266258.php.

Nordqvist, Joseph. 2017. "Apples: Health Benefits, Facts, Research." Medical News Today. MediLexicon International. April 11. https://www.medicalnewstoday.com/articles/267290.php.

Nordqvist, Joseph. 2017. "Oregano: Health Benefits, Uses, and Side Effects." Medical News Today. MediLexicon International. December 11. http://www.medicalnewstoday.com/articles/266259.php.

"The Nutrition of Clams / Nutrition / Healthy Eating." 2018. Nutrition. Accessed July 18. https://www.fitday.com/fitness-articles/nutrition/healthy-eating/the-nutrition-of-clams.html.

"Omega-3 Fatty Acids." 2018. University of Maryland Medical System. Accessed July 18. https://www.umms.org/ummc/patients-visitors/health-library/medical-encyclopedia/images/omega3-fatty-acids.

Pagán, Camille Noe. 2018. "Herbs and Spices for Your Health: Ginger, Turmeric, Cinnamon, and More." WebMD. WebMD. Accessed July 18. https://www.webmd.com/healthy-aging/over-50-nutrition-17/spices-and-herbs-health-benefits.

"Papaya." 2018. Cabbage. Accessed July 18. http://www.whfoods.com/genpage.php?tname=foodspice&dbid=47.

Paravantes, Elena. 2015. "Top 5 Health Benefits of Olive Oil." Olive Oil Times. Olive Oil Times. October 21. http://www.oliveoiltimes.com/olive-oil-health-news/top-5-health-benefits-of-olive-oil/31463/3.

Pattani, Aneri. 2016. "America Is Suddenly Losing the Battle against Its No. 1 Killer Disease." CNBC. CNBC. December 22. https://www.cnbc.com/2016/12/22/as-heart-disease-deaths-rise-health-experts-focus-on-prevention.html.

Phillip, John. 2011. "Naturalnews.com Printable Article." NaturalNews. September 29. http://www.naturalnews.com/z033722_zinc_memory.html.

"Phytosterols, Sterols & Stanols." 2018. Cleveland Clinic. Accessed July 18. https://my.clevelandclinic.org/health/articles/17368-phytosterols-sterols--stanols.

Presse, N, S Belleville, P Gaudreau, C E Greenwood, M J Kergoat, J A Morais, H Payette, B Shatenstein, and G Ferland. 2013. "Vitamin K Status and Cognitive Function in Healthy Older Adults." Neurobiology of Aging 34 (12): 2777–83. doi:10.1016/j.neurobiolaging.2013.05.031.

"Quercetin: Uses, Side Effects, Interactions, Dosage, and Warning." 2018. WebMD. WebMD. Accessed July 18. http://www.webmd.com/vitamins-supplements/ingredientmono-294-quercetin.aspx?activeingredientid=294&activeingredientname=quercetin.

Reinagel, Monica. 2014. "What Are Phytosterols?" Scientific American. July 16. https://www.scientificamerican.com/article/what-are-phytosterols/.

Richards, Byron J. 2018. "Vitamin K Improves Cognitive Function." Wellness Resources. Accessed July 19. https://www.wellnessresources.com/news/vitamin-k-helps-cognitive-function.

Roizman, Tracey. 2017. "What Are the Health Benefits of Eating Chestnuts?" Livestrong.com. Leaf Group. October 3. http://www.livestrong.com/article/470050-what-are-the-health-benefits-of-eating-chestnuts/.

Saba. 2018. "10 Amazing Health Benefits Of Blue Cheese." STYLECRAZE. IncnutIncnut. Accessed July 18. https://www.stylecraze.com/articles/amazing-health-benefits-of-blue-cheese/.

Shilhavy, Brian. 2015. "Coconut Oil and Alzheimer's." Coconut Oil. January 12. http://coconutoil.com/coconut-oil-alzheimers/.

"Spice of Life: 7 Surprising Health Benefits of Curry Powder." 2018. Benenden Health. Accessed July 18. https://www.benenden.co.uk/be-healthy/nutrition/spice-of-life-7-surprising-health-benefits-of-curry-powder/.

Spritzler, Franziska. 2018. "8 Health Benefits of Eating Nuts." Healthline. Healthline Media. Accessed July 18. https://www.healthline.com/nutrition/8-benefits-of-nuts.

Spritzler, Franziska. 2018. "Ghee: Is It Even Better Than Regular Butter?" Healthline. Healthline Media. Accessed July 18. https://www.healthline.com/nutrition/ghee.

"Strawberries." 2018. Cabbage. Accessed July 18. http://www.whfoods.com/genpage.php?tname=foodspice&dbid=32.

"Stroke." 2017. Centers for Disease Control and Prevention. Centers for Disease Control and Prevention. September 6. https://www.cdc.gov/stroke/facts.htm.

"Suggested Servings from Each Food Group." 2017. How Cigarettes Damage Your Body. July 20. http://www.heart.org/HEARTORG/HealthyLiving/HealthyEating/HealthyDietGoals/Suggested-Servings-from-Each-Food-Group_UCM_318186_Article.jsp#.W0-3Oy_MzVo.

Szalay, Jessie. 2017. "Watermelon: Health Benefits, Risks & Nutrition Facts." LiveScience. Purch. May 10. https://www.livescience.com/46019-watermelon-nutrition.html.

Tadimalla, Ravi Teja. 2018. "14 Amazing Health Benefits Of Macadamia Nuts." STYLECRAZE. IncnutIncnut. June 1. http://www.stylecraze.com/articles/amazing-health-benefits-of-macadamia-nuts/.

Taub-Dix, Bonnie. 2014. "11 Health Benefits Of Beans." *The Huffington Post*. TheHuffingtonPost.com. November 17. https://www.huffingtonpost.com/2012/08/16/beans-health-benefits_n_1792504.html.

Thomson, Julie R. 2017. "The Best Salad Greens, Ranked By Nutrition." *The Huffington Post*. TheHuffingtonPost.com. September 8. www.huffingtonpost.com/entry/best-salad-greens-nutrition_us_59aedc1ae4b0b5e531014eb8.

Tidy, Colin. 2016. "Health Benefits of a Mediterranean Diet | Heart Disease." Patient.info. Patient.info. June 20. http://www.patient.co.uk/health/Health-Benefits-of-the-Mediterranean-Diet.

Torrens, Kerry. 2018. "The Health Benefits of Nuts." BBC Good Food. Accessed July 19. http://www.bbcgoodfood.com/howto/guide/health-benefits-nuts.

Tremblay, Sylvie. 2018. "What Do Oats Do for the Body?" Healthy Eating | SF Gate. June 11. https://healthyeating.sfgate.com/oats-body-2593.html.

Villines, Zawn. 2018. "9 Health Benefits of Beans." Medical News Today. MediLexicon International. Accessed July 18. https://www.medicalnewstoday.com/articles/320192.php.

Ware, Megan. 2017. "Pineapple: Health Benefits, Recipes, Health Risks." Medical News Today. MediLexicon International. January 6. http://www.medicalnewstoday.com/articles/276903.php.

Ware, Megan. 2017. "Mushrooms: Nutritional Value and Health Benefits." Medical News Today. MediLexicon International. February 23. https://www.medicalnewstoday.com/articles/278858.php.

Ware, Megan. 2017. "Watermelon: Health Benefits, Nutrition, and Risks." Medical News Today. MediLexicon International. June 20. http://www.medicalnewstoday.com/articles/266886.php.

Ware, Megan. 2017. "Chia Seeds: Health Benefits and Recipe Tips." Medical News Today. MediLexicon International. August 2. https://www.medicalnewstoday.com/articles/291334.php.

Ware, Megan. 2017. "Mangoes: Health Benefits, Nutrition, Recipes." Medical News Today. MediLexicon International. August 22. http://www.medicalnewstoday.com/articles/275921.php.

Ware, Megan. 2017. "Sweet Potatoes: Health Benefits and Nutritional Information." Medical News Today. MediLexicon International. September 1. https://www.medicalnewstoday.com/articles/281438.php.

Ware, Megan. 2017. "Blueberries: Health Benefits, Facts, and Research." Medical News Today. MediLexicon International. September 5. http://www.medicalnewstoday.com/articles/287710.php.

Ware, Megan. 2017. "12 Health Benefits of Avocado." Medical News Today. MediLexicon International. September 12. https://www.medicalnewstoday.com/articles/270406.php#Possible health benefits of avocados.

Ware, Megan. 2017. "Bananas: Health Benefits, Tips, and Risks." Medical News Today. MediLexicon International. November 28. http://www.medicalnewstoday.com/articles/271157.php.

Ware, Megan. 2017. "Mint: Benefits, Diet, Risks, and Nutrition." Medical News Today. MediLexicon International. December 11. http://www.medicalnewstoday.com/articles/275944.php.

Ware, Megan. 2017. "Peaches: Benefits, Nutrition, Dietary Tips, and Risks." Medical News Today. MediLexicon International. December 20. http://www.medicalnewstoday.com/articles/274620.php.

Ware, Megan. 2018. "Lemons: Benefits, Nutrition, Tips, and Risks." Medical News Today. MediLexicon International. January 5. http://www.medicalnewstoday.com/articles/283476.php.

Ware, Megan. 2018. "Pumpkins: Health Benefits and Nutritional Breakdown." Medical News Today. MediLexicon International. January 5. https://www.medicalnewstoday.com/articles/279610.php.

Ware, Megan. 2018. "Raspberries: Health Benefits, Nutrition, Dietary Tips, and Risks." Medical News Today. MediLexicon International. January 5. http://www.medicalnewstoday.com/articles/283018.php.

Ware, Megan. 2018. "Brussels Sprouts: Health Benefits and Nutritional Information." Medical News Today. MediLexicon International. January 19. https://www.medicalnewstoday.com/articles/284765.php.

Ware, Megan. 2018. "Fennel: Health Benefits and Dietary Tips." Medical News Today. MediLexicon International. January 23. https://www.medicalnewstoday.com/articles/284096.php.

West, Helen. 2017. "5 Health Benefits of Greek Yogurt." EcoWatch. EcoWatch. February 19. https://www.ecowatch.com/health-benefits-greek-yogurt-2265934371.html.

"What Is Dragon Fruit Good For?" 2018. Mercola.com. Accessed July 18. https://foodfacts.mercola.com/dragon-fruit.html.

"What Is Ghee?" 2018. What Is Ghee. Accessed July 18. http://whatisghee.com/.

"What Is Ghee and Is It Really Better than Butter?" 2018. MyRecipes. Accessed July 18. http://www.myrecipes.com/special-diet/what-is-ghee.

"Why Americans Love Sandwiches." 2014. Gunther Toody's. September 15. https://gunthertoodys.com/why-americans-love-sandwiches/.

"Why Do We Need Minerals. Why Do We Need to Eat Minerals?" 2018. Eat Balanced. Accessed July 18. http://www.eatbalanced.com/why-eat-balanced/why-do-we-need-minerals/.

Wilcox, Julie. 2012. "7 Health Benefits of Lentils." Mindbody green. mindbodygreen. July 17. https://www.mindbodygreen.com/0-5488/7-Health-Benefits-of-Lentils.html.

Wolk, Victoria. 2018. "Here's How Much You Need To Exercise To Prevent Alzheimer's." Prevention. Prevention. May 25. http://www.prevention.com/fitness/how-exercise-can-help-prevent-alzheimers-disease.

"The Women's Alzheimer's Movement." 2018. The Women's Alzheimers Movement. Accessed July 18. http://thewomensalzheimersmovement.org/.

Zelman, Kathleen M. 2018. "6 Best Foods You're Not Eating." WebMD. WebMD. Accessed July 18. https://www.webmd.com/diet/features/best-foods-you-are-not-eating#3.

Zelman, Kathleen M. 2018. "The Many Benefits of Breakfast." WebMD. WebMD. Accessed July 18. https://www.webmd.com/diet/features/many-benefits-breakfast#1.

About the Author

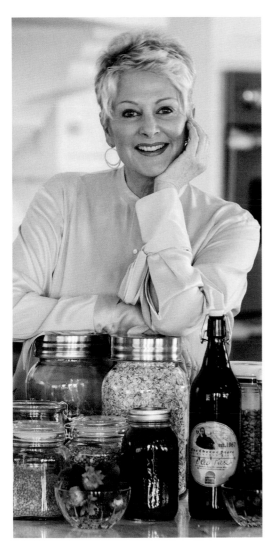

Cristina Ferrare is the author of two *New York Times* bestselling books and was featured in a series of cooking segments on Oprah.com entitled *Cooking with Cristina*. She began her career as a model and graced the covers of every major fashion magazine, including *Vogue*, *Harper's Bazaar*, and *Cosmopolitan*. Cristina co-hosted *AM Los Angeles*, the highest-rated morning television show during her five-year tenure, and also hosted *Cristina and Friends* and *Home and Family*. She was a substitute co-host on *Good Morning America* and co-hosted with Regis Philbin on *Live! with Regis and Kathie Lee*. Her primetime series for CBS, *Shame on You*, was one of the first magazine format shows that featured consumer fraud and awareness. Cristina is also an entrepreneur whose successful lifestyle home décor company—Ferrare With Company—is distributed in the U.S. and overseas. She blogs about health and cooking as well.